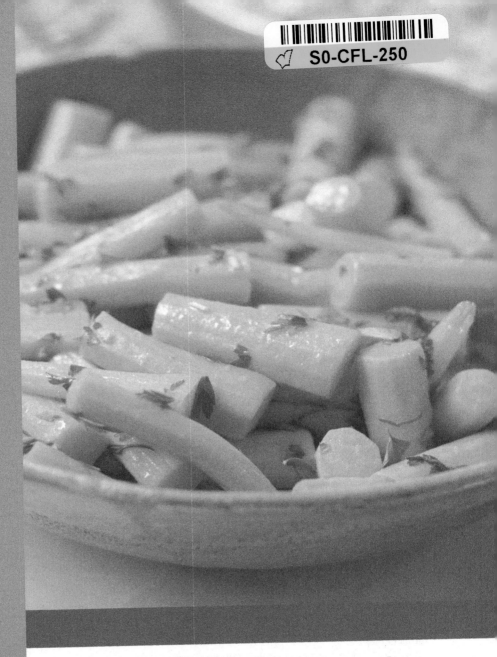

Vegetable Recipes for Coumadin® Users

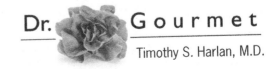

Dr. Gourmet

Timothy S. Harlan, M.D.

Vegetable Recipes for Coumadin Users

Terms of Use
The Content of this book and the Dr. Gourmet website, including recipes, nutrition and health information, text, graphics, images, calculators, columns and other material contained on the Dr. Gourmet website or in this book, is solely for informational purposes. Any communication with any staff member of the Dr. Gourmet website does not constitute a physician or health care provider / patient relationship.

Information on the Dr. Gourmet website or in this book should not be used in place of a visit or call to your doctor. You should not make changes in your medical therapy or any advice given to you by your physician without consulting them first.

The Content presented on the Dr. Gourmet website and in this book is not intended to be a substitute for professional medical advice. No effort is made at diagnosis or treatment of any condition. Only your doctor can help you with diagnosis and treatment of medical problems. Always discuss your concerns with your physician, asking any questions you may have regarding your medical condition. Do not disregard any advice given to you by any medical professional because of any information that you have read on the Dr. Gourmet website or in this book.

Table of Contents

Introduction

Coumadin® (warfarin) is a prescription medication used for anticoagulation. It is often referred to as "a blood thinner," but that is not really an accurate description. It works by inhibiting enzymes that lead to blood clotting. It is a well researched, effective oral medication. (Other brand names for warfarin are Jantoven, Marevan, and Waran.)

Its primary use is to treat or prevent blood clots. When the blood clots in a vein or artery, physicians refer to it as a *thrombus*. When the thrombus breaks free and travels to other parts of the body it is known as an *embolus*. A common problem known as deep vein thrombosis (DVT) occurs when such clots form in the large veins in the legs or arms. These will commonly form and then break free and travel to the lungs, blocking blood flow, which is known as a pulmonary embolus (PE).

Other uses include:
- ✔ Pulmonary embolism
- ✔ Artificial heart valves
- ✔ Atrial fibrillation
- ✔ Atrial flutter
- ✔ Transient ischemic attacks (TIAs)
- ✔ Stroke
- ✔ Heart attack
- ✔ Blockages of the arteries
- ✔ After some surgeries
- ✔ Those with disorders of the clotting system

How it Works

Warfarin is a synthetic version of a class of chemicals known as coumarins. These are found in many plants, such as woodruff, lavender and licorice. It was named by combining the acronym for the Wisconsin Alumni Research Foundation (WARF) and the suffix for coumarin (arin). The Foundation provided the original research grants, and it was indeed originally developed as rat poison, but is seldom used as a rat poison today because similar but much more potent forms are now available for that purpose.

Warfarin's anticoagulant effect works because the drug inhibits production of proteins known as "clotting factors." These proteins are produced in the liver and are dependent on an adequate supply of Vitamin K. The clotting factor proteins are the foundation of the "intrinsic" clotting pathway. There are many proteins that work together, and warfarin blocks four of them: Factors VII, IX, X, and II. Creation of these proteins in the liver is dependent on Vitamin K, which can come from dietary sources but can also be created by bacteria in the large intestine. After being absorbed, Vitamin K is stored in the liver. Consequently Vitamin K is the vital regulatory step for the production of the clotting Factors VII, IX, X, and II.

Warfarin blocks the action of Vitamin K within the liver by blocking the absorption sites in the liver needed for the uptake of Vitamin K. With the lowered ability for Vitamin K absorption, there is reduced production of the clotting factors. Consequently, dietary intake of Vitamin K affects the effectiveness of warfarin.

Prescribing Coumadin® (warfarin)

Doctors prescribe Coumadin to patients who are prone to thrombosis and also to prevent them in those who have already formed blood clots. There are numerous conditions that can lead to clot formation, including prosthetic heart valves, atrial fibrillation, deep venous thrombosis and pulmonary embolism. There are also those with inherited problems with clotting factors, like antiphospholipid syndrome and factor five leiden, for whom we prescribe warfarin to prevent clotting. Sometimes the drug is used after myocardial infarction (heart attack) and stroke.

Finding the correct dose of warfarin for patients is complicated by the fact that it interacts with many other over-the-counter and prescription medications, as well as supplements. This interaction can cause Coumadin to be more or less effective. The activity of the drug has to be monitored by frequent blood testing for the international normalized ratio (INR). If the INR is high, the dose is too high. Conversely, if the INR is too low, the medication dose needs to be increased. (We used to use a test, the Prothrombin Time, sometimes called the "Pro Time" or PT, but its accuracy varied between labs. Now results are standardized through the use of the INR.)

Adjusting the Dose

It is very important that you always know when will be your next blood test for the INR. It is equally important to know what dose you are taking. It's a good idea to keep a warfarin calendar to help you keep track. Get a small calendar and carry it with you (in your wallet or purse). Write your doses of warfarin in the appropriate days until the next blood test. When you take your dose, circle that day so that you know you have taken it. In the day scheduled for your blood test, write "Get INR" to remind yourself. After the test, if you have not heard from your doctor's office about your results, call them for any new instructions.

The target level of the INR will depend on why you are taking warfarin. In most cases the target range for INR is 2.0-3.0. In some cases, however, the range is higher. Your doctor will set the target based on your particular condition.

Most physicians prefer for their patients to take warfarin in the evening. This is primarily because blood tests are typically taken in the morning, and it will give your doctor time to contact you after your INR is checked. He or she can then change the dose, if needed, before you take your evening medication. There are now home testing kits available and insurance companies are paying for these more and more. Check with your doctor and your insurance company to see if you qualify.

You **must** tell **any** doctor who prescribes medicine for you that you are taking warfarin. If you have any unusual bleeding let your doctor know right away. Call your doctor with any questions or issues earlier rather than later. It's a good idea to have a "Medic Alert" bracelet stating that you are taking warfarin.

Interactions

Taking other medications can also increase the risk of bleeding. The most common are antiplatelet drugs such as aspirin, clopidogrel or nonsteroidal anti-inflammatory drugs like ibuprofen (Advil) or naproxyn (Aleve, Naprosyn).

There are many other drug-to-drug interactions, and because of genetic factors the body's processing of the drug can vary widely between patients.

Excessive alcohol use can also affect how warfarin is processed in the liver and elevate the INR. Most physicians will caution patients about the use of alcohol while taking warfarin. Commonly doctors will allow a few drinks after INR is stable.

Foods that are high in Vitamin K have also been reported to interact with warfarin. Visit DrGourmet.com/shop for our book, *Vitamin K Levels in Common Foods,* which includes over 800 common foods and their exact Vitamin K content in micrograms.

Supplements

Warfarin also interacts with many herbs, including (but not limited to):

- ✔ Ginkgo Biloba
- ✔ St. John's Wort
- ✔ American Ginseng
- ✔ Garlic as a supplement (not fresh garlic)

Vitamin K Dosage

I get the question all the time about how much Vitamin K is right for folks taking Coumadin® (warfarin). Unfortunately, there's no perfect study to guide just how much Vitamin K is too much for those taking Coumadin. Most physicians recommend limiting foods that contain very high or even moderate amounts of Vitamin K. At the same time, there's never been a recommendation to severely limit Vitamin K intake.

The Recommended Daily Allowance (RDA) for Vitamin K is 80 micrograms (mcg) for males and 70 mcg for females. The majority of ingredients contain small amounts - in the under 15 mcg range - so keeping an eye on foods that contain more than 20 - 25 mcg per serving is a good rule of thumb.

Avoiding **all** Vitamin K might be just as much of a problem as getting too much, however. Studies have clearly shown that eating foods that are higher in Vitamin K will have an effect on the effectiveness of Coumadin and the INR. Most people who either take warfarin themselves or those who help patients manage their anti-coagulation know this, but there is some research now that shows eating too little Vitamin K can have the same effect.

So what to do? How much is too much? How little is too little? It appears, from what research we have, that in those folks who were taking Coumadin, 29 mcg was too little and **76 mcg just right** to keep their INR stable.

While it's not a perfect way to look at the issue of how much is too much Vitamin K in the diet for warfarin users, another study showed an effect on the INR in those taking 150 - 200 mcg per day in Vitamin K supplements. These are the levels found in Vitamin K rich foods such as spinach, collard greens and broccoli.

For the number of folks who use this medication and the fact that there's no great replacement on the horizon, it is a shame that a large study has not been done to help answer this question more clearly. For the time being, we have to be content with the small studies that point toward an optimum near the RDA guidelines for Vitamin K.

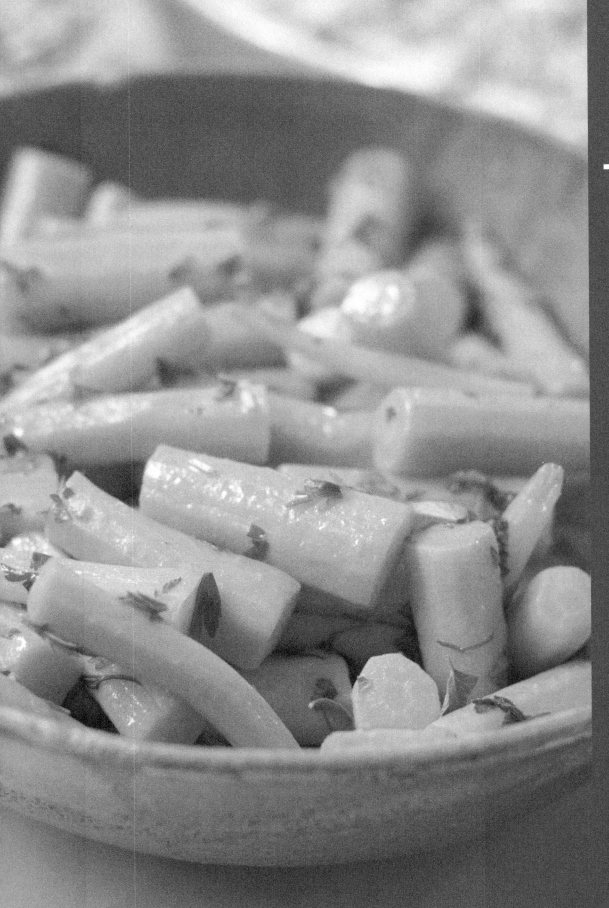

Baked Potato

Servings = 1
Serving size = 1 6-ounce potato

This recipe can easily be multiplied but does not make very good leftovers.

1	6 ounce Idaho potato

Preheat the oven to 325°F.

Scrub the potato and place in the oven. Bake for 30 to 40 minutes until the potato gives slightly when you squeeze it.

"A satisfied customer-we should have him stuffed!"
Basil Fawlty, Owner, Fawlty Towers

The refrigerator light goes on...
I do love baked potatoes. They're so simple but there are so many different ways to cook them. The main decision is whether to wrap or not. Foil traps the moisture and the potato steams along with baking making for a moister flesh. I prefer to not wrap potatoes and bake them unwrapped. The skin turns out crispy and the flesh fluffier I feel.

Idaho potatoes are the best for baking. You can bake waxy potatoes like Yukon gold or red potatoes but they will not have the same fluffiness as Idahos. If you are in a hurry, the microwave will cook your potato but these dry out too much. You can cook it for 2 minutes on high prior to putting the potato in the oven and it will preheat the potato and shorten the cooking time by about 10 minutes. Of course, the Nutrition Facts don't include what you put on top of your potato. Loading it down with butter will add a lot of calories. I like a little bit of salt and pepper with sour cream and maybe some grated cheddar cheese.

Nutrition Facts

Serving Size	1 6-ounce Idaho potato
Servings	1
Calories 156	Calories from Fat 2
	(% Daily Value)
Total Fat 0 g	(0 %)
Saturated Fat 0 g	(0 %)
Trans Fat 0 g	
Monounsaturated Fat 0 g	
Cholesterol 0 mg	(0 %)
Sodium 17 mg	(1 %)
Total Carbohydrates 36 g	(12 %)
Dietary Fiber 4 g	(15 %)
Sugars 2 g	
Protein 4 g	
Vitamin A 0 %	Vitamin C 27 %
Calcium 3 %	Iron 10 %
Vitamin K3 mcg	
Potassium 899 mg	Magnesium 47 mg

Baked Sweet Potato

Servings = 1
Serving size = one 6-ounce yam

This recipe can easily be multiplied as many times as you like. This recipe does not make very good left-overs.

1	6-ounce yam
1 tsp	unsalted butter
1/2 ounce	goat cheese
	sprinkle salt

Wash the yam well.

Place the yam on a sheet of aluminum foil and place in the oven. Set the temperature to 325°F.

Bake the potato for about 40 minutes until it is soft. You'll know because it will give slightly when squeezed.

Serve with the butter and goat cheese. Sprinkle just a tiny bit of salt over the top.

"We must eat to live and live to eat."
Henry Fielding, Playwright

The refrigerator light goes on...
More and more yams are being sold in America as yams. For the longest time they would be labeled "sweet potatoes." Actual sweet potatoes are not widely available.

So why not call this recipe "Baked Yam"? I don't know. Baked Sweet Potato just sounds better.

Nutrition Facts

Serving size	1 6-ounce yam
Servings	1
Calories 273	Calories from Fat 64
	(% Daily Value)
Total Fat 7g	(11%)
Saturated Fat 4g	(19%)
Trans Fat 0 g	
Monounsaturated Fat 2g	
Cholesterol 17mg	(5%)
Sodium 213mg	(8%)
Total Carbohydrates 47g	(18%)
Dietary Fiber 7g	(24%)
Sugars 1g	
Protein 6g	
Vitamin A 11%	Vitamin C 48%
Calcium 2%	Iron 8%
Vitamin K 4 mcg	
Potassium 1393 mg	Magnesium 38 mg

Black Eyed Peas

Servings = 6
Serving size = 1 cup

"Do Southerners laugh at different things than Northerners do? Yes--Northerners."
Roy Blount, Humorist

This recipe can easily be multiplied or may be divided by 2. This recipe is better if made the night before and it keeps well for about 48 hours in the fridge.

3 quarts	water
2 1/3 cups	dried black eyed peas
1 tsp	canola or grapeseed oil
1 ounce	lean ham
1 medium	onion
2	ribs celery
6 cups	water
3/4 tsp	salt
1/8 tsp	fresh ground black pepper

The refrigerator light goes on...
You wouldn't think that black eyed peas are all that good for you but they are. The cheap, lowly black eye is a member of the legume family and chock full of everything good for you. A great ingredient as a side dish with your Oven Fried Chicken or used in a salad.

Rinse the peas well and place in a large pot. Cover with cold water and soak for at leas an hour (overnight if possible). Drain the peas.

** Canned no salt added black eyed peas may be used. Rinse well. You will need two 15 ounce cans for this recipe. Drain and rinse the canned beans well. **

Place a large sauce pan over medium heat. Add the oil and lean ham. Cook until the ham is browned well.

Add the onion and celery and cook for about 5 minutes stirring frequently.

** If you are using canned beans start with only three cups of water and add more as needed.

Add the black eyed peas, water, salt and pepper. Reduce the heat to medium-low and cook for about two hours until the beans are tender. You may need more water during cooking.

** If you are using canned beans the cooking process will take an hour at the most.

Nutrition Facts

Serving Size	1 cup	
Servings	6	
Calories 126	Calories from Fat 14	
	(% Daily Value)	
Total Fat 2 g	(3 %)	
Saturated Fat 0 g	(2 %)	
Trans Fat 0 g		
Monounsaturated Fat 0 g		
Cholesterol 3 mg	(1 %)	
Sodium 367 mg	(15 %)	
Total Carbohydrates 21 g	(7 %)	
Dietary Fiber 6 g	(38 %)	
Sugars 4 g		
Protein 8 g		
Vitamin A 1 %	Vitamin C 5 %	
Calcium 3 %	Iron 13 %	
Vitamin K 6 mcg		
Potassium 325 mg	Magnesium 51 mg	

Blue Cheese Acorn Squash

Servings = 2
Serving size = 1/2 small acorn squash

This recipe can easily be multiplied. This recipe makes OK leftovers. Reheat carefully.

1	small acorn squash (about 1 1b.)
	spray olive oil
1 1/2 ounces	blue cheese (crumbled)

Preheat the oven to 325°F.

Cut the squash in half and scoop out the seeds.

Spray a large skillet lightly with olive oil. Place the squash in the skillet cut side down and place the pan in the oven. Roast for about 35 – 40 minutes.

Remove the squash and let cool slightly. Slice as thinly as possible into crescents. Divide the crescents onto two oven proof plates or au gratin dishes. Arrange the crescents so that they overlap slightly.

Sprinkle the blue cheese across the top distributing the cheese evenly. Place the plates in the oven for about 5 minutes until the cheese is melted.

"Strange to see how a good dinner and feasting reconciles everybody."
Samuel Pepys, Diarist

The refrigerator light goes on...
This is one of those deceptively simple recipes that is so good. A bit of squash and a bit of cheese... cooking is supposed to be harder than this. Sometimes it is just this easy and delicious.

Nutrition Facts

Serving Size	1/2 small acorn squash
Servings	2
Calories 164	Calories from Fat 55
	(% Daily Value)
Total Fat 6 g	(10 %)
Saturated Fat 2 g	(10 %)
Trans Fat 0 g	
Monounsaturated Fat 2 g	
Cholesterol 16 mg	(5 %)
Sodium 300 mg	(12 %)
Total Carbohydrates 24 g	(8 %)
Dietary Fiber 3 g	(13 %)
Sugars 0 g	
Protein 6 g	
Vitamin A 20 %	Vitamin C 41 %
Calcium 18 %	Iron 9 %
Vitamin K 0 mcg	
Potassium 831 mg	Magnesium 77 mg

Candied Carrots

Servings = 2
Serving size = about one cup carrots

This recipe can easily be multiplied. This recipe does not make very good leftovers.

2 cups	water
8 ounces	carrots (peeled and sliced)
1 Tbsp.	light spread
1 Tbsp.	maple syrup
1/4 tsp.	salt

Place the water in a pot fitted with a steamer basket over high heat. Steam for about 10-15 minutes until the carrots are slightly tender.

Combine the cooked carrots with the light spread, maple syrup and salt and serve.

"An intellectual carrot. The mind boggles."
Lederer and Nyby, Screenwriters of
The Thing from Another World

The refrigerator light goes on...
Most candied carrots recipes are way too sweet and the amount of brown sugar or molasses or maple syrup masks the flavor of the carrots. The combination of the light spread and a small amount of maple syrup with the salt balances nicely with the natural sweetness of the carrots.

Nutrition Facts

Serving size	about 1 cup carrots
Servings	4
Calories 96	Calories from Fat 26
	(% Daily Value)
Total Fat 3g	(4%)
Saturated Fat 1g	(4%)
Trans Fat 0 g	
Monounsaturated Fat 1g	
Cholesterol 0mg	(0%)
Sodium 276mg	(11%)
Total Carbohydrates 18g	(6%)
Dietary Fiber 3g	(13%)
Sugars 11g	
Protein 1g	
Vitamin A 391%	Vitamin C 11%
Calcium 4%	Iron 3%
Vitamin K 17 mcg	
Potassium 387 mg	Magnesium 15 mg

Cheese Stuffed Peppers

Servings = 2
Serving size = 1 pepper

This recipe can easily be multiplied by 2 or 3. This recipe does not make very good leftovers.

2	bell peppers (yellow, red, or orange)
2 ounces	goat cheese
1/4 Cup	cilantro leaves
	spray olive oil

Preheat the oven to 325°F.

Place the peppers in the oven and roast for about 20 - 25 minutes. Turn the peppers about 1/4 turn about every 5 minutes so that they roast evenly on all sides.

While the peppers are cooling place the goat cheese in a bowl and add the chopped cilantro. Mix together until well blended.

Remove and let cool on the counter. Slice into the pepper lengthwise on one side and remove the seeds.

Place 1/4 of the goat cheese mixture inside each half of the roasted pepper. Fold over and press slightly so that the cheese flattens out inside the pepper.

Preheat the oven again to 325°F. Place a medium skillet in the oven and when hot spray lightly with olive oil. Add the peppers and return the pan to the oven and cook for about 7 - 10 minutes until they are hot and serve.

"Some writers say the leaves [cilantro] are used for seasoning, but this statement seems odd, as all the green parts of the plant exhale a very strong odor of the wood-bug, whence the Greek name of the plant."

Vilmorin-Andrieux,
19th Century Writer

The refrigerator light goes on...
This is a quick and simple and so tasty side dish for any spicy meal. Almost any herb will do - if you're making Spanish food, use thyme and oregano, or for Southwestern or Mexican the cilantro works great. Basil is fantastic as well.

Nutrition Facts

Serving size	1 pepper
Servings	2

Calories 108	Calories from Fat 54
	(% Daily Value)
Total Fat 6 g	(10 %)
Saturated Fat 4 g	(21 %)
Trans Fat g	
Monounsaturated Fat 1 g	
Cholesterol 13 mg	(4 %)
Sodium 109 mg	(5 %)
Total Carbohydrates 8 g	(3 %)
Dietary Fiber 3 g	(11 %)
Sugars 4 g	
Protein 7 g	
Vitamin A 21 %	Vitamin C 221 %
Calcium 6 %	Iron 6 %
Vitamin K 19 mcg	
Potassium 305 mg	Magnesium 21 mg

Corn and Parsnip Puree

Servings = 4
Serving size = about 1 cup

This recipe can easily be multiplied and makes great leftovers.

3 tsp	olive oil (divided)
1 small	white onion (diced)
12 ounce	parsnips (peeled and diced)
2 cups	water
1/4 tsp	salt
1/2 tsp	marjoram
1 ounce	reduced fat cream cheese
2	ears corn (kernels cut from cob) (about 3 cups)
to taste	fresh ground black pepper

Place 2 teaspoons of the olive oil in a medium sauce pan over medium high heat. Add the onion and cook for about 3 minutes, stirring occasionally.

Add the parsnips and cook for about 2 minutes. Add the water and the salt. Cover and reduce the heat to medium so that the parsnips are simmering. Cook for about 20 minutes, stirring occasionally, until the parsnips are soft. Remove from the heat and stir in the marjoram and cream cheese.

Allow the cream cheese to melt, then let cool slightly and then crush with a fork until smooth.

While the parsnips are cooling, place the other teaspoon of olive oil in a large skillet over medium high heat. Cook, tossing almost continuously, until the corn begins to brown. Add the pepper and cook for about 8 to 10 minutes total.

Add the pureed parsnips and cook for about a minute until heated through. Serve.

"The President cannot make clouds to rain and cannot make the corn to grow, he cannot make business good; although when these things occur, political parties do claim some credit for the good things that have happened in this way."
William Howard Taft,
American President

The refrigerator light goes on...
These two are perfect together. Sweet and creamy parsnips and sweet corn kernels make the perfect side dish, especially with fish and chicken.

Nutrition Facts

Serving size	about 1 cup
Servings	4
Calories 110	Calories from Fat 38 **(% Daily Value)**
Total Fat 4 g	(7 %)
Saturated Fat 1 g	(3 %)
Trans Fat 0g	
Monounsaturated Fat 4 g	
Cholesterol 0 mg	(0 %)
Sodium 159 mg	(7 %)
Total Carbohydrates 18 g	(6 %)
Dietary Fiber 3 g	(11 %)
Sugars 4 g	
Protein 3 g	
Vitamin A 0 %	Vitamin C 13 %
Calcium 1 %	Iron 3 %
Vitamin K 4 mcg	
Potassium 266 mg	Magnesium 33 mg

Cowboy Pinto Beans

Servings = 4
Serving size = about 1 1/4 cup

This recipe can easily be multiplied up to 8 times. This recipe will keep well in the refrigerator for 3-4 days. Reheat gently. (Also good cold.)

1 tsp	canola or olive oil
1 medium	white onion (diced)
1 medium	green bell pepper (diced)
2 15 ounce cans	no salt added pinto beans (drained and rinsed)
2 cups	water
1 Tbsp	tomato paste
1 Tbsp	molasses
1 tsp	chili powder
1/2 tsp	salt
to taste	fresh ground black pepper
1/2 tsp	cumin

Place the oil in a pan over medium-high heat. Add the onion and sauté for three minutes. Add the bell pepper and cook for another two minutes.

Add the beans, water, tomato paste, molasses, chili powder, salt, pepper and cumin and stir. Cook on medium high for about 5 minutes.

Reduce the heat and simmer on low for about 45 minutes or until the sauce thickens. Stir them occasionally while they are simmering.

Serve.

"I always wanted to be a cowboy, and Jedi Knights are basically cowboys in space, right?"
Liam Neeson, Actor

The refrigerator light goes on...
The key is to cook the beans fast for about ten minutes on medium-high heat. Stir them often in that first ten minutes and then reduce the heat to very low and simmer, covered. Stir them only occasionally. The stirring will break up a few beans and help thicken the sauce.

Nutrition Facts

Serving size	about 1 1/4 cup
Servings	4

Calories 129	Calories from Fat 15
	(% Daily Value)
Total Fat 2 g	(3 %)
Saturated Fat 0 g	(1 %)
Trans Fat 0 g	
Monounsaturated Fat 1 g	
Cholesterol 0 mg	(0 %)
Sodium 305 mg	(2 %)
Total Carbohydrates 23 g	(8 %)
Dietary Fiber 7 g	(27 %)
Sugars 4 g	
Protein 6 g	
Vitamin A 7 %	Vitamin C 43 %
Calcium 5 %	Iron 11 %
Vitamin K 6 mcg	
Potassium 466 mg	Magnesium 51 mg

Creamed Corn

Servings = 2
Serving size = about 1 cup

This recipe can easily be multiplied. This recipe does OK as leftovers. Reheat gently.

1 tsp.	canola oil
1/2 medium	white onion (minced)
2 tsp.	all purpose flour
2 ears	corn (cut off cob)
1/4 tsp.	salt
1/2 cup	2% milk
1 cup	water
to taste	fresh ground black pepper

Heat the canola oil in a medium sized skillet over medium heat.

Add the minced onion and cook for about 3 - 5 minutes until they begin to soften.

Add the flour one teaspoon at a time until it is well blended into the onions.

Add the corn kernels and cook for about 3 minutes stirring frequently. Add the salt, milk, water and pepper.

Cook over medium heat simmering for about 20 minutes stirring frequently.

Place the mixture in a strainer over a medium bowl. When all of the liquids have drained through add half of the corn. Using a blender or stick blender, puree until smooth and add the mixture back to the skillet with the remaining corn.

Reheat gently while stirring. Serve.

"Then plough deep while sluggards sleep, and you shall have corn to sell and to keep."
Benjamin Franklin, Genius

The refrigerator light goes on...
I love creamed corn, but most recipes are really high in fat and / or salt. It depends on whether you buy frozen or canned or make your own, but most all of them are just over the top nutritionally. This recipe gives you so much of what I love in creamed corn: fresh corn flavor, sweetness and (best of all) creaminess. Serve this with any comfort food you choose.

Nutrition Facts

Serving size	1 cup
Servings	2
Calories 153	Calories from Fat 40
	(% Daily Value)
Total Fat 5 g	(7 %)
Saturated Fat 1 g	(6 %)
Trans Fat 0 g	
Monounsaturated Fat 2 g	
Cholesterol 5 mg	(2 %)
Sodium 342 mg	(14 %)
Total Carbohydrates 25 g	(8 %)
Dietary Fiber 3 g	(12 %)
Sugars 7 g	
Protein 6 g	
Vitamin A 0 %	Vitamin C 15 %
Calcium 10 %	Iron 4 %
Vitamin K 2 mcg	
Potassium 404 mg	Magnesium 47 mg

Cumin, Black Eyes and Corn Salad

Servings = 6
Serving size = about 1 cup

This recipe can easily be multiplied. This recipe makes great leftovers. Cooking time does not include chilling time.

"Well, they're Southern people, and if they know you are working at home they think nothing of walking right in for coffee. But they wouldn't dream of interrupting you at golf."
Harper Lee, Author

	spray olive oil
1/3 cup	raw pecan pieces
2 large	ears corn (cut kernels from ears)
2 15 ounce cans	no salt added black eyed peas (drained and rinsed)
1 small	shallot (minced)
1/2	red bell pepper (seeded and diced)
3/4 tsp	salt
to taste	fresh ground black pepper
2 tsp	ground cumin
1 Tbsp	olive oil
1 Tbsp	maple syrup

The refrigerator light goes on...
The cumin in these black eyes adds just the zing to complement the sweetness of the peas and roasted corn.

Place a large non-stick skillet over high heat. Spray lightly with oil.

Add the pecans. After about 90 seconds they will begin to toast. Cook, tossing frequently, for about 2 – 3 minutes until they begin to brown.

Add the corn kernels and cook, tossing frequently, for about 5 – 8 minutes. If the corn browns too fast, reduce the heat to medium-high.

Place the cooked corn in a medium mixing bowl with the black eyed peas, shallot, red pepper, salt, pepper, cumin, olive oil and maple syrup.

Fold together well and chill for at least two hours before serving.

Nutrition Facts

Serving size	about 1 cup
Servings	6
Calories 204	Calories from Fat 64
	(% Daily Value)
Total Fat 8 g	(12%)
Saturated Fat 1 g	(4 %)
Trans Fat 0 g	
Monounsaturated Fat 4 g	
Cholesterol 41 mg	(14 %)
Sodium 301 mg	(1 %)
Total Carbohydrates 28 g	(9 %)
Dietary Fiber 7 g	(29 %)
Sugars 6 g	
Protein 8 g	
Vitamin A 9 %	Vitamin C 26 %
Calcium 4 %	Iron 17 %
Vitamin K 4 mcg	
Potassium 404 mg	Magnesium 68 mg

Curried Roasted Squash

Servings = 2
Serving size = 1 large squash

his recipe make great leftovers and works in salads and sandwiches.

1 lb.	yellow squash (sliced in half lengthwise)
1 tsp.	olive oil
1/8 tsp.	salt
1/4 tsp.	curry powder
to taste	fresh ground black pepper

Preheat the oven to 325°F. Place a large skillet in the oven.

When the pan is hot place the olive oil in the skillet and then add the squash, cut side down.

Place the pan in the oven and roast for about twenty minutes. Shake the pan occasionally to keep the squash from sticking.

Turn the squash over and sprinkle the salt, curry powder and pepper over the top. Return the pan to the oven and cook for another 5 to 7 minutes.

"So far as I am able to judge, nothing has been left undone, either by man or nature, to make India the most extraordinary country that the sun visits on his rounds. Nothing seems to have been forgotten, nothing overlooked."

Mark Twain, American Genius

The refrigerator light goes on...
This recipe is super simple and the curried squash comes out of the oven tasting as though you put butter on it. This is a great side dish with almost any main course.

Nutrition Facts

Serving size	1 large squash
Servings	2
Calories 64	Calories from Fat 25
	(% Daily Value)
Total Fat 3 g	(4 %)
Saturated Fat <1 g	(1 %)
Trans Fat 0 g	
Monounsaturated Fat 2 g	
Cholesterol 0 mg	(0 %)
Sodium 150 mg	(6 %)
Total Carbohydrates 9 g	(3 %)
Dietary Fiber 4 g	(16 %)
Sugars 0 g	
Protein 2 g	
Vitamin A 8 %	Vitamin C 32 %
Calcium 8 %	Iron 8 %
Vitamin K 1 mcg	
Potassium 485 mg	Magnesium 49 mg

Dill Pesto

Servings = 6
Serving size = 2 Tablespoons

This recipe can easily be multiplied by 2. This dill
pesto keeps well for up to a week in the refrigerator.

2 Tbsp	pine nuts
2 cloves	garllc (minced)
4 cups	fresh dill
1 ounce	Parmigiano-Reggiano (grated)
2 Tbsp	water
2 tsp	fresh lemon juice
2 Tbsp	extra virgin olive oil

Combine pine nuts, garlic fresh dill, parmesan, water,
lemon juice and olive oil in blender and blend until
smooth.

Chill thoroughly.

"Pesto is the quiche of the 80's."
Nora Ephron, Playwright

The refrigerator light goes on...
I think that most of the pesto that I am served is
simply greasy. It almost always has too much olive
oil and then the sauce separates. Good cooking is
about a balance of flavors and not using fat or salt
to hide the sins of poor recipes.

Nutrition Facts

Serving size	2 Tablespoons
Servings	6
Calories 92	Calories from Fat 76
	(% Daily Value)
Total Fat 9 g	(14%)
Saturated Fat 2 g	(8 %)
Trans Fat 0 g	
Monounsaturated Fat 5 g	
Cholesterol 3 mg	(1 %)
Sodium 76 mg	(3 %)
Total Carbohydrates 1 g	(0 %)
Dietary Fiber 1 g	(0 %)
Sugars 0 g	
Protein 2 g	
Vitamin A 9 %	Vitamin C 9 %
Calcium 7%	Iron 4 %
Vitamin K 5 mcg	
Potassium 78 mg	Magnesium 16 mg

Eggplant Pesto

Servings = 6
Serving size = about 1/2 cup

This recipe can be multiplied up to 5 times. This recipe keeps well for about 72 hours in the fridge.

	spray olive oil
1 lb	eggplant (sliced in half lengthwise)
1/2 cup	walnut pieces
1/4 cup	basil leaves
3 Tbsp	olive oil
2 cloves	garlic (minced)
1 ounce	Parmigiano-Reggiano (grated)
1 tsp	white wine vinegar
1/4 tsp	salt

Preheat the oven to 325°F. Spray a large skillet with oil and place the eggplant in the pan cut side down.

Place the pan in the oven and let the eggplant roast about 30 minutes until tender. Remove and let cool.

While the eggplant is cooling, place the walnuts, basil, olive oil, garlic, Parmigiano-Reggiano, vinegar, salt and pepper in a blender and puree.

When the eggplant is cool, scrape the eggplant out of the skin and add it to the blender. Discard the skin. Puree until smooth.

"How can people say they don't eat eggplant when God loves the color and the French love the name? I don't understand."

Jeff Smith, The Frugal Gourmet

The refrigerator light goes on...
I love the aroma and flavor of roasted eggplant. When I was working on this recipe my wife said, "Hey, let's just eat it now," as it came out of the oven. She's right. A little sprinkle of salt, a bit of pepper and some olive oil, and that's living. But I digress.

You can use this Eggplant Pesto in place of any other pesto, but it's more subtle so you'll need more. Where about two or so tablespoons of a Basil Pesto would be enough in a pasta dish, this works great as a sauce and you can use about a half cup or so.

This is just as versatile as any other pesto. You can use it in pasta, as a spread on sandwiches or bruschetta. It also works great in making hors d'oeuvres and other appetizers. A dollop in a creamy soup would be perfect.

Nutrition Facts

Serving size	about 1/2 cup
Servings	6
Calories 162	Calories from Fat 131
	(% Daily Value)
Total Fat 14 g	(23 %)
Saturated Fat 3 g	(12 %)
Trans Fat 0 g	
Monounsaturated Fat 8 g	
Cholesterol 3 mg	(1 %)
Sodium 176 mg	(7 %)
Total Carbohydrates 6 g	(3 %)
Dietary Fiber 4 g	(10 %)
Sugars 3 g	
Protein 4 g	
Vitamin A 0 %	Vitamin C 3 %
Calcium 7 %	Iron 2 %
Vitamin K 8 mcg	
Potassium 222 mg	Magnesium 28 mg

French Fries

Servings = 4
Serving size = about 4 ounces fries

This recipe can easily be multiplied by 2, but must be cooked in two batches. These do not keep very well at all.

1 lb	russet potatoes
1 quart	chilled water
1	tray ice cubes
1/2 tsp	salt
	spray canola oil

After the potatoes are peeled and sliced, place them in a mixing bowl with cold water and ice cubes. Soak for 30 minutes.

Preheat oven to 400°F.

After soaking the potatoes, drain them and then pat dry with a paper towel.

Place the potatoes and salt in a zipper bag. Spray the potatoes for about three seconds with the canola oil and seal the zipper bag. Shake to coat the potatoes well with the oil and salt.

Carefully place the potatoes on a non-stick cookie sheet. Avoid the fries touching each other. Spray lightly with the canola oil.

Place the cookie sheet in the oven and allow the potatoes to bake for about 7 minutes. Turn the potatoes at least twice, cooking for about 7 minutes after each turn. Total cooking time will be 20 – 25 minutes.

Serve immediately.

"Zen... does not confuse spirituality with thinking about God while one is peeling potatoes. Zen spirituality is just to peel the potatoes"
Alan W. Watts, *The Way of Zen*

The refrigerator light goes on...
Oven fried foods are just like deep-fried ones, if you handle them right. Most of the time you have to eat the dish right away. These French Fries, for instance, will keep for all of about 20 minutes (about the amount of time as ones that have been deep fried).

Nutrition Facts

Serving size	about 4 ounces fries
Servings	4
Calories 86	Calories from Fat 1
	(% Daily Value)
Total Fat 0 g	(0 %)
Saturated Fat 0 g	(0 %)
Trans Fat 0 g	
Monounsaturated Fat 0 g	
Cholesterol 0 mg	(0 %)
Sodium 297 mg	(12 %)
Total Carbohydrates 20 g	(7 %)
Dietary Fiber 2 g	(10 %)
Sugars 2 g	
Protein 1 g	
Vitamin A 0 %	Vitamin C 37 %
Calcium 1 %	Iron 5 %
Vitamin K 2 mcg	
Potassium 472 mg	Magnesium 26 mg

Green Beans Almondine

Servings = 2
Serving size = about 1 cup beans

This recipe can easily be multiplied. This recipe makes good leftovers. Serve chilled or reheat very gently.

1 quart	water
1 lb.	green beans
1 tsp.	olive oil
1 tsp.	unsalted butter
1 Tbsp.	sliced almonds
1/8 tsp.	salt
to taste	fresh ground black pepper

Place the water in a large skillet pot over high heat. When the water is at a shiver (almost boiling) add the green beans.

Cook them for about 5 - 7 minutes and remove them from the pan to a strainer or a paper towel.

Heat the olive oil and butter in a medium skillet over medium heat. Add the sliced almonds. Cook gently, stirring frequently, until the almonds begin to brown. If they seem to be browning too fast reduce the heat.

Add the green beans, salt and pepper. Cook, tossing frequently, for about another 2 - 3 minutes and serve.

"Training is everything. The peach was once a bitter almond; cauliflower is nothing but cabbage with a college education."
Mark Twain, Author

The refrigerator light goes on...
We used to call these string beans or snap beans when I was a kid because you had to snap the tip off and peel the string away from the pod. These days the beans have been bred to not have strings that need removing.

Green beans are a legume and there's no doubt that they are good for you. There's a lot of Vitamin C, but look at that fiber. That's as much as 2 slices of some whole wheat breads and this has about a third of the calories.

You can use good old fashioned green beans (snap beans) or the skinny little French style beans (haricot vert). I like pole beans - the large flat green bean - but these are not as available in the grocery as much as they once were. Look for them in the late summer at your farmer's market.

Nutrition Facts

Serving size	about 1 cup beans
Servings	4
Calories 87	Calories from Fat 49
	(% Daily Value)
Total Fat 6 g	(9 %)
Saturated Fat 2 g	(8 %)
Trans Fat 0 g	
Monounsaturated Fat 3 g	
Cholesterol 5 mg	(2 %)
Sodium 158 mg	(7 %)
Total Carbohydrates 9 g	(3 %)
Dietary Fiber 4 g	(17 %)
Sugars 2 g	
Protein 3 g	
Vitamin A 17 %	Vitamin C 30 %
Calcium 5 %	Iron 7 %
Vitamin K 18 mcg	
Potassium 254 mg	Magnesium 35 mg

Green Beans with Garlic and Ginger

Servings = 2
Serving size = 4 ounces green beans

This recipe can easily be multiplied. This recipe makes great leftovers. Serve chilled or reheat very gently.

2 tsp	sesame oil
1 clove	garlic (minced)
2 tsp	fresh ginger (minced)
8 ounces	fresh whole green beans
2 Tbsp	water
2 tsp	low sodium soy sauce
to taste	fresh ground black pepper

Place the olive oil in a large skillet over medium heat.

Add the garlic and ginger. Cook, stirring frequently, for about 1 minute.

Add the green beans and toss well.

Reduce the heat to medium-low, add the water and cover the pan. Cook for about 10 to 15 minutes, tossing occasionally.

Add the soy sauce and pepper. Cook uncovered for another minute and serve.

"Without garlic I simply would not care to live."
Louis Diat, Chef

The refrigerator light goes on...
The water helps the green beans to steam, but it isn't so much that they will get soggy. At the end of the cooking, when adding the soy sauce and pepper, increasing the heat to medium high will help evaporate any extra liquid.

Garlic and ginger combine with the soy sauce for a wonderful Asian flavor. Simple ingredients, great results.

Nutrition Facts

Serving size	4 ounces green beans
Servings	2
Calories 82	Calories from Fat 42
	(% Daily Value)
Total Fat 5 g	(7 %)
Saturated Fat <1 g	(3 %)
Trans Fat 0 g	
Monounsaturated Fat 2 g	
Cholesterol 0 mg	(0 %)
Sodium 184 mg	(7 %)
Total Carbohydrates 8 g	(4 %)
Dietary Fiber 4 g	(12 %)
Sugars 2 g	
Protein 2 g	
Vitamin A 16 %	Vitamin C 33 %
Calcium 5 %	Iron 9 %
Vitamin K 17 mcg	
Potassium 261 mg	Magnesium 31 mg

Green Beans with Red Onion

Servings = 4
Serving size = 4 ounces green beans

This recipe can easily be multiplied. These keep well for about 48 hours in the fridge and is good served cold at picnics.

1 quart	water
1 lb.	green beans (trim the ends)
2 Tbsp.	light spread (like Promise Buttery Spread Light)
1/4 cup	red onion (diced)
1/4 tsp.	salt
1 tsp.	fresh thyme leaves
to taste	fresh ground black pepper

Place the water in a large stock pot over high heat. When the water is at a slow boil reduce the heat until the water shivers. Add the green beans and blanch for about 7 - 10 minutes until al dente.

While the beans are cooking place a large skillet over medium heat. Add the spread and as it melts toss in the red onion. Cook slowly and reduce the heat if the onion is turning brown. Stir frequently.

When the beans are done remove them from the blanching water and shake off the excess water. Add them to the red onions with the salt, thyme and black pepper.

Cook over medium heat for about two minutes and serve.

Add ground black pepper to taste.

"Most people call the 'accompaniments'; just as a hat, handbag, or briefcase is to the suit, so vegetables are to the main dish."
Graham Kerr, Genius

The refrigerator light goes on...
Beans are so delicious and so good for you. These green beans will work with many different herbs; I like the taste of the thyme, however. Rosemary is wonderful as is a touch of jasmine. If you don't have the red onion, shallot will work. (White onions are fine but I like the touch of color.)

Nutrition Facts

Serving size	4 ounces green beans
Servings	4
Calories 64	Calories from Fat 25
	(% Daily Value)
Total Fat 3 g	(4 %)
Saturated Fat <1 g	(1 %)
Trans Fat 0 g	
Monounsaturated Fat 2 g	
Cholesterol 0 mg	(0 %)
Sodium 150 mg	(6 %)
Total Carbohydrates 9 g	(3 %)
Dietary Fiber 4 g	(16 %)
Sugars 0 g	
Protein 2 g	
Vitamin A 8 %	Vitamin C 32 %
Calcium 8 %	Iron 8 %
Vitamin K 1 mcg	
Potassium 485 mg	Magnesium 49 mg

Guacamole

Servings = 8
Serving size = about 3 tablespoons

This recipe can easily be multiplied and keeps well, refrigerated, for about 48 hours.

16 ounces	avocado
2 Tbsp	red onion (diced)
4 ounces	tomato (coarsely chopped)
1/4 cup	cilantro leaves (chopped)
1/2 tsp	cumin
1/8 tsp	cayenne pepper
1 Tbsp	fresh lime juice
1/2 tsp	salt
to taste	fresh ground black pepper

Place the avocado, onion, tomato, cilantro, cumin, cayenne, salt and pepper in a bowl.

Using a fork, mash the guacamole until blended and the avocado is coarse chunks. Chill for about an hour.

"Training is everything. The peach was once a bitter almond; cauliflower is nothing but cabbage with a college education."
Mark Twain, Author

The refrigerator light goes on...
Ah... avocados. I love them and they are best in guacamole with other bright flavors like the tomato and cilantro. You can make it as spicy as you like, but I like mine mild so that I can taste all the ingredients.

The avocados should be just right – not too firm and not too soft. If you purchase them firm, place the avocado in a paper bag on the counter and close the top. After a day or so they'll be just right.

Nutrition Facts

Serving size	about 3 tablespoons
Servings	8
Calories 95	Calories from Fat 69
	(% Daily Value)
Total Fat 8 g	(13 %)
Saturated Fat 1 g	(6 %)
Trans Fat 0 g	
Monounsaturated Fat 6 g	
Cholesterol 0 mg	(0 %)
Sodium 151 mg	(6 %)
Total Carbohydrates 6 g	(2 %)
Dietary Fiber 4 g	(16 %)
Sugars 1 g	
Protein 1 g	
Vitamin A 5 %	Vitamin C 14 %
Calcium 1 %	Iron 3 %
Vitamin K 15 mcg	
Potassium 320 mg	Magnesium 19 mg

Herbed Zucchini

Servings = 4
Serving size = about 2/3 cup

This recipe can easily be multiplied using a large skillet. This recipe does not make very good leftovers.

1 Tbsp.	olive oil
1 lb.	zucchini (cut into 1/4 inch dice)
2 Tbsp.	fresh herbs of your choice (minced)
1/4 tsp.	salt
to taste	fresh ground black pepper

Place the olive oil in a large non-stick skillet over medium-high heat. When the oil is hot, add the zucchini. Let the zucchini cook without stirring for about 3 minutes. If it appears to be cooking too fast, reduce the heat to medium.

Toss the zucchini well and cook for about 7 - 10 more minutes. As the cubes begin to brown, add the herbs, salt and pepper and continue to toss.

Do not over cook the zucchini. As soon as the outside is lightly browned and it is slightly soft, serve.

"If one consults enough herbals...every sickness known to humanity will be listed as being cured by sage."
Varro Taylor, Ph.D., Pharmacologist

The refrigerator light goes on...
The choice of herbs here is not important. Use what you have in the garden or the fridge. Equal amounts of basil, chive, sage, rosemary and oregano will do, but you could just as easily choose thyme, sage, marjoram and tarragon. This recipe will work with dried herbs, but it just isn't quite as good somehow.

Nutrition Facts

Serving size	about 2/3 cup
Servings	4
Calories 51	Calories from Fat 32
	(% Daily Value)
Total Fat 4 g	(6 %)
Saturated Fat 1 g	(3 %)
Trans Fat 0 g	
Monounsaturated Fat 3 g	
Cholesterol 0 mg	(0 %)
Sodium 88 mg	(4 %)
Total Carbohydrates 5 g	(2 %)
Dietary Fiber 2 g	(7 %)
Sugars 2 g	
Protein 2 g	
Vitamin A 6 %	Vitamin C 33 %
Calcium 4 %	Iron 8 %
Vitamin K 26 mcg	
Potassium 321 mg	Magnesium 23 mg

Honey Peas

Servings = 2
Serving size = about 1 cup

This recipe can easily be multiplied. This recipe does not make very good leftovers.

1 cup	frozen peas
1 tsp.	olive oil
1 tsp.	honey
1/8 tsp.	salt
to taste	fresh ground black pepper

Place the peas in a small sauce pan over medium heat.

When the peas are hot, add the butter, olive oil, honey, salt and pepper. Cook until all of the water is evaporated. Serve.

"I always eat my peas with honey: I've done it all my life. They do taste kind of funny but it keeps them on my knife."

Winnie the Pooh

The refrigerator light goes on...
Just a touch of olive oil and honey makes simple frozen peas rich and elegant. Super simple and really delicious. I like to add a lot of pepper to this – it really spices it up.

Nutrition Facts

Serving size	1 cup
Servings	2
Calories 69	Calories from Fat 22
	(% Daily Value)
Total Fat 2 g	(4 %)
Saturated Fat 0 g	(2 %)
Trans Fat 0 g	
Monounsaturated Fat 2 g	
Cholesterol 0 mg	(0 %)
Sodium 103 mg	(4 %)
Total Carbohydrates 10 g	(3 %)
Dietary Fiber 2 g	(9 %)
Sugars 5 g	
Protein 3 g	
Vitamin A 21 %	Vitamin C 15 %
Calcium 1 %	Iron 4 %
Vitamin K 15 mcg	
Potassium 78 mg	Magnesium 13 mg

Jalapeno Mashed Potatoes

Servings = 2
Serving size = about 1 cup

This recipe can easily be multiplied but does not make good leftovers.

2 quarts	water
8 ounces	red potatoes
1 ounce	reduced-fat Monterey Jack cheese
2 Tbsp	non-fat buttermilk
2 tsp	reduced-fat sour cream
1/4 tsp	salt
to taste	fresh ground black pepper
2 tsp	pickled jalapeno

Place the water in a large stock pot over high heat.

Quarter the potatoes and add to the stock pot. Cover with water by about an inch. Bring to boil and then reduce heat until the water is simmering.

Cook the potatoes about 15 – 20 minutes until slightly soft in the middle. They should give when squeezed.

Remove from heat and drain water. Add cheese, buttermilk, sour cream, salt, pepper and minced jalapeno. Mash potatoes until creamy.

I like to leave some chunks in my potatoes. If you like them smooth it is best to use a potato ricer because over mashing will result in pasty potatoes.

"This is a great German potato ricer. It's good and solid. You see, the potato goes in and you go schoooom and out she comes! I love great big things like this, it really works very well. Of course it all comes apart for washing, so it's a very practical instrument."

Julia Child, Genius

The refrigerator light goes on...
You can use fresh jalapeno with this as well, mincing it finely. There's a slightly different flavor between the fresh and pickled, with the fresh being spicier. If you do use fresh, begin with less – maybe only a teaspoon - and adjust for flavor. The potatoes shouldn't be so spicy as to overpower any dish you might serve with them.

Nutrition Facts

Serving size	about 1 cup
Servings	2
Calories 147	Calories from Fat 36
	(% Daily Value)
Total Fat 4 g	(6 %)
Saturated Fat 2 g	(12 %)
Trans Fat 0 g	
Monounsaturated Fat 1 g	
Cholesterol 12 mg	(4 %)
Sodium 489 mg	(20 %)
Total Carbohydrates 20 g	(7 %)
Dietary Fiber 2 g	(8 %)
Sugars 3 g	
Protein 8 g	
Vitamin A 6 %	Vitamin C 39 %
Calcium 16 %	Iron 6 %
Vitamin K 4 mcg	
Potassium 604 mg	Magnesium 34 mg

Jicama Slaw

Servings = 6
Serving size = about 1 cup

"Orange is the happiest color."
Frank Sinatra

This recipe can easily be multiplied and is actually better the second day.

1 1/2 lbs.	jicama (peeled and matchstick)
2	satsumas (tangerines) (peeled and sectioned)
1/4 cup	dried pepitas (pumpkin seeds)
1/2 tsp.	lime zest
1	lime (juiced)
1/2 tsp.	salt
to taste	fresh ground black pepper
1 tsp.	honey
1/4 cup	fresh cilantro

The refrigerator light goes on...
Jicama makes a great base for a salad. It is slightly sweet and slightly crunchy and it can go in so many ways – savory, sweet, spicy or even tart.

Cut each section of the satsumas in half.

Place the jicama, satsumas, pepitas, lime zest, lime juice, salt, pepper, honey and cilantro in a large bowl and fold together.

Refrigerate until time to serve.

Nutrition Facts

Serving size	about 1 cup
Servings	6
Calories 97	Calories from Fat 26
	(% Daily Value)
Total Fat 3 g	(4 %)
Saturated Fat <1 g	(2 %)
Trans Fat 0 g	
Monounsaturated Fat 1 g	
Cholesterol 0 mg	(0 %)
Sodium 201 mg	(8 %)
Total Carbohydrates 17 g	(5 %)
Dietary Fiber 7 g	(23 %)
Sugars 6 g	
Protein 2 g	
Vitamin A 4 %	Vitamin C 58 %
Calcium 1 %	Iron 9 %
Vitamin K 4 mcg	
Potassium 279 mg	Magnesium 50 mg

Mashed Yams

Servings = 4
Serving size = about 1 cup

This recipe can easily be multiplied. This recipe
makes good leftovers and will keep well in the refrigerator for about 48 hours. Reheat gently.

1 quart	water
1 lb	yams (peeled and cubed)
1 tsp	extra virgin olive oil
1 large	shallot (minced)
1/4 tsp	dried rosemary
1/4 tsp	salt
to taste	fresh ground black pepper
2 Tbsp	light spread (like Promise Buttery Spread Light or Smart Balance Light)
1/4 cup	non-fat buttermilk
2 Tbsp	2% milk

Place the water in a large stock pot fitted with a
steamer basket over high heat.

Add the cubed yams to the steamer basket and steam
until they break slightly with a fork.

While the yams are cooking, place the olive oil in
a small skillet over medium heat. Add the shallots
and rosemary and cook gently until the shallots are
softened.

Place the cooked yams together with the shallot and
rosemary mixture in a bowl. Add the salt, pepper,
spread and buttermilk and mash with a fork until
smooth. Add the 2% milk slowly as the yams are
mashed smooth.

The mashed yams can be reheated gently in a microwave.

*"Strange to see how a good dinner and feasting
reconciles everybody."*

Samuel Pepys, Culinarian

The refrigerator light goes on...
This is the perfect recipe to substitute for mashed
potatoes. The same creamy mashed potato dish
that's so comforting with the twist of added flavor.
And the added benefit of more fiber!

Nutrition Facts

Serving size	about 1 cup
Servings	4
Calories 188	Calories from Fat 37
	(% Daily Value)
Total Fat 4 g	(6 %)
Saturated Fat 1 g	(5 %)
Trans Fat 0 g	
Monounsaturated Fat 2 g	
Cholesterol 1 mg	(0 %)
Sodium 215 mg	(9 %)
Total Carbohydrates 35 g	(12 %)
Dietary Fiber 5 g	(19 %)
Sugars 2 g	
Protein 3 g	
Vitamin A 14 %	Vitamin C 35 %
Calcium 6 %	Iron 4 %
Vitamin K 6 mcg	
Potassium 1021 mg	Magnesium 31 mg

Mashed Yams with Mint

Servings = 2
Serving size = about 1 1/2 cups

This recipe can easily be multiplied and can be divided by 2, but it does not make very good leftovers.

10 ounces	yams
1/8 tsp	salt
6 large	fresh mint leaves (minced)
1 tsp	unsalted butter
2 Tbsp	reduced fat sour cream
1 tsp	maple syrup
to taste	fresh ground black pepper

Preheat the oven to 325°F.

Place the yams in the oven and roast for about 40 minutes.

Remove the yams and place in a bowl with the salt, mint, butter, sour cream, maple syrup and pepper.

Using a fork, mash the yams until smooth and blended with the other ingredients.

"Every cloud has its silver lining, but it is sometimes a little difficult to get it to the mint."
Don Marquis, Writer

The refrigerator light goes on...
I love plain mashed yams, but the hint of peppermint makes these sweet and savory and a bit spicy.

Nutrition Facts

Serving size	about 1 1/2 cups
Servings	2
Calories 231	Calories from Fat 35
	(% Daily Value)
Total Fat 4 g	(6 %)
Saturated Fat 2 g	(12 %)
Trans Fat 0 g	
Monounsaturated Fat 1 g	
Cholesterol 13 mg	(4 %)
Sodium 168 mg	(7 %)
Total Carbohydrates 47 g	(16 %)
Dietary Fiber 6 g	(23 %)
Sugars 8 g	
Protein 3 g	
Vitamin A 8 %	Vitamin C 40 %
Calcium 6 %	Iron 5 %
Vitamin K 3 mcg	
Potassium 1196 mg	Magnesium 31 mg

Minted Cucumbers

Servings = 2
Serving size = about 1 cup

This recipe can easily be multiplied but does not make very good leftovers.

2 medium	cucumbers (peeled, seeded & sliced into crescents)
2 tsp.	olive oil
2 Tbsp.	rice vinegar
1/8 tsp.	salt
to taste	fresh ground black pepper
1/4 tsp.	dried peppermint

Fold together the cucumbers, olive oil, rice vinegar, salt, pepper and peppermint.

Chill.

"People mature with age and experience. I hope I more resemble a fine wine than bad vinegar."
Rick Kaplan, Television executive

The refrigerator light goes on...
I have loved cucumbers in vinegar since I was a kid. My mother made them very simply as peeled and sliced cucumbers (not seeded) with oil, white vinegar and a bit of salt and pepper. The mint was sprinkled on sometimes since it grew wild in our side yard. A taste of the South in the summer.

This variation is a little more elegant, and I like to use rice vinegar because it's not as acidic and lets the sweetness of the cucumber and mint come through better.

Nutrition Facts

Serving size	about 1 cup
Servings	2
Calories 68	Calories from Fat 43
	(% Daily Value)
Total Fat 5 g	(7 %)
Saturated Fat 1 g	(3 %)
Trans Fat 0 g	
Monounsaturated Fat 3 g	
Cholesterol 0 mg	(0 %)
Sodium 150 mg	(6 %)
Total Carbohydrates 5 g	(2 %)
Dietary Fiber 1 g	(6 %)
Sugars 3 g	
Protein 1 g	
Vitamin A 4 %	Vitamin C 11 %
Calcium 3 %	Iron 3 %
Vitamin K 17 mcg	
Potassium 288 mg	Magnesium 26 mg

Mustard Vinaigrette Green Beans

Servings = 3
Serving size = about 1 cup

This recipe can easily be multiplied but does not keep well.

1 quart	water
12 ounces	green beans
2 tsp.	olive oil
1 tsp.	balsamic vinegar
2 tsp.	Dijon mustard
2 tsp.	water
1/4 tsp.	salt
to taste	fresh ground black pepper
1/8 tsp	dried tarragon

Place the water in a medium pot, fitted with a steamer basket, over high heat.

Add the green beans and cover. Cook for about 10 minutes until tender.

While the beans are cooking, place the olive oil, vinegar, mustard, water, salt, pepper and tarragon in a medium mixing bowl. Whisk until smooth.

When the beans are tender add them to the dressing. Toss to coat well. Serve.

"Love is like a mustard seed; planted by God and watered by men.

Muda Saint Michael, Poet

The refrigerator light goes on...
There's enough sauce to make this simple side dish rich and tasty. When I asked my wife to taste these she said, "Wow, that's the stuff." We both had to tear ourselves away from the bowl (not that it matters all that much since there's almost no calories).

Nutrition Facts

Serving size	1 cup
Servings	3
Calories 64	Calories from Fat 29
	(% Daily Value)
Total Fat 3 g	(5 %)
Saturated Fat 0 g	(2 %)
Trans Fat 0 g	
Monounsaturated Fat 2 g	
Cholesterol 0 mg	(0 %)
Sodium 239 mg	(10 %)
Total Carbohydrates 8 g	(3 %)
Dietary Fiber 4 g	(16 %)
Sugars 2 g	
Protein 2 g	
Vitamin A 16 %	Vitamin C 31 %
Calcium 4 %	Iron 7 %
Vitamin K 18 mcg	
Potassium 240 mg	Magnesium 30 mg

Paprika Potatoes

Servings = 4
Serving size = about 1 cup

This recipe can easily be multiplied by 2. This recipe can be easily doubled using a large roasting pan. Left-over potatoes, cold, make great additions to salads or may be reheated gently.

1 lb	small red or Yukon gold
potatoes	
2 tsp	olive oil
1 clove	garlic (minced)
1 tsp	paprika
1/4 tsp	salt
to taste	fresh ground black pepper

Place a large skillet in the oven and preheat to 375° F.

Add the olive oil and garlic to the hot pan.

Add the potatoes and toss to coat with the oil.

Sprinkle the paprika, salt and pepper over the potatoes and toss.

Place the pan in the oven, reduce the heat to 325°F.

Roast the potatoes for about 20 minutes. Toss them about every five minutes to brown on all sides. Serve when the potatoes are tender.

"If the divine creator has taken pains to give us delicious and exquisite things to eat, the least we can do is prepare them well and serve them with ceremony."

Fernand Point, 20th century French chef

The refrigerator light goes on...
I especially like this recipe using fingerling potatoes. They are now often as inexpensive as regular potatoes. I slice them in half lengthwise if they are small and quarter them lengthwise if they are larger.

Nutrition Facts

Serving size	about 1 cup
Servings	4
Calories 102	Calories from Fat 22
	(% Daily Value)
Total Fat 2 g	(4 %)
Saturated Fat <1 g	(6 %)
Trans Fat 0 g	
Monounsaturated Fat 2 g	
Cholesterol 0 mg	(0 %)
Sodium 152 mg	(6 %)
Total Carbohydrates 18 g	(8 %)
Dietary Fiber 2 g	(9 %)
Sugars 1 g	
Protein 2 g	
Vitamin A 5 %	Vitamin C 18 %
Calcium 0 %	Iron 5 %
Vitamin K 4 mcg	
Potassium 531 mg	Magnesium 26 mg

Parmesan Squash

Servings = 2
Serving size = 1 large squash

This recipe can easily be multiplied. This recipe does not make very good leftovers.

2 large	yellow squash (8 ounces each)
2 cups	water
to taste	fresh ground black pepper
2 Tbsp.	fresh herbs of your choice (minced)
1 ounce	Parmigiano-reggiano (grated)

Place the water in a medium pot fitted with a steamer basket over high heat.

Preheat the oven to 325°F.

Cut about 1/4 inch from the stem end of the squash and then slice lengthwise. Place the four halves in the steamer and steam until slightly tender.

Remove the steamed squash and place in a shallow baking dish. Place the dish in the oven and cook for about 10 minutes. Remove and sprinkle with pepper, fresh herbs and equal amounts of Parmigiano-reggiano.

Return the pan to the oven and cook until the parmesan is melted (about 5 minutes).

"There's no sauce in the world like hunger."
Miguel de Cervantes, Author

The refrigerator light goes on...
These are two perfect ingredients that make a wonderful dish. The yellow squash tastes like summer and its own buttery flavor is enhanced by the parmesan. I especially like using just a little bit of rosemary for the herb.

Nutrition Facts

| Serving size | 1 large squash |
| Servings | 2 |

Calories 99	Calories from Fat 37
	(% Daily Value)
Total Fat 4 g	(7 %)
Saturated Fat 2 g	(10) %
Trans Fat 0 g	
Monounsaturated Fat 1 g	
Cholesterol 10 mg	(3 %)
Sodium 233 mg	(10 %)
Total Carbohydrates 10 g	(3 %)
Dietary Fiber 4 g	(17 %)
Sugars 0 g	
Protein 7 g	
Vitamin A 8 %	Vitamin C 32 %
Calcium 22 %	Iron 7 %
Vitamin K 0 mcg	
Potassium 497 mg	Magnesium 54 mg

Parsnip French Fries

Servings = 4
Serving size = about 4 ounces fries

This recipe can easily be multiplied but must be cooked in two batches.

1 lb.	parsnips
1 quart	chilled water
1 tray	ice cubes
1/8 tsp.	salt
1/8 tsp.	dried rosemary
to taste	fresh ground black pepper
	spray olive oil

Peel the parsnips and cut lengthwise into the shape of thick French fries.

Place them in a mixing bowl with cold water and ice cubes. Soak for 30 minutes.

Preheat oven to 400°F.

After soaking the parsnips, drain them and then pat dry with a paper towel.

Place the parsnips and salt in a zipper bag with the rosemary and pepper. Spray the parsnips for about three seconds with the oil and seal the zipper bag. Shake to coat the potatoes well with the oil and salt.

Carefully place the parsnips on a non-stick cookie sheet. Avoid the fries touching each other. Spray lightly with the oil.

Place the cookie sheet in the oven and allow the parsnips to bake for about 7 minutes. Turn the parsnips at least twice, cooking for about 7 minutes after each turn. Total cooking time will be 20 – 25 minutes.

Serve immediately.

""Zen. . . does not confuse spirituality with thinking about God while one is peeling potatoes. Zen spirituality is just to peel the potatoes."
Alan W. Watts, The Way of Zen

The refrigerator light goes on...
These are a great alternative to French Fries (even the Dr. Gourmet oven baked version). They have about 3 times the fiber of fries using potatoes and are sweet and delicious. The rosemary, olive oil and pepper give them a fantastic flavor but you could use almost any herb or spice that appeals to you.

Oven fried foods are just like deep-fried ones, if you handle them right. Most of the time, you have to eat the dish right away. These Parsnip French Fries, for instance, will keep for all of about 20 minutes (about the amount of time as ones that have been deep fried).

Nutrition Facts

Serving size	about 4 ounces fries
Servings	4

Calories 95	Calories from Fat 13
	(% Daily Value)
Total Fat 1.5 g	(2 %)
Saturated Fat 0 g	(0 %)
Trans Fats 1 g	
Monounsaturated Fat 0 g	
Cholesterol 0 mg	(0 %)
Sodium 84 mg	(12 %)
Total Carbohydrates 20 g	(8 %)
Dietary Fiber 6 g	(20 %)
Sugars 6 g	
Protein 2 g	
Vitamin A 0 %	Vitamin C 32 %
Calcium 4 %	Iron 4 %
Vitamin K 26 mcg	
Potassium 425 mg	Magnesium 33 mg

Plain Mashed Potatoes

Servings = 4
Serving size = about 1 cup

This recipe can be multiplied but does not keep well.

3 quarts	water
1 lb	Yukon Gold potatoes
2 tsp	unsalted butter
1/4 cup	non-fat buttermilk
1/4 cup	2% milk
1/4 tsp	salt
	fresh ground black pepper

Place the water in a large stock pot over high heat.

Quarter the potatoes and add to the stock pot. Cover with water by about an inch. Bring to boil and then reduce heat until the water is simmering.

Cook the potatoes about 15 – 20 minutes until slightly soft in the middle. They should give when squeezed.

Remove from heat and drain water. Add butter, buttermilk, milk and salt. Mash potatoes until creamy. I like to leave some chunks. If you like them smooth be careful because over mashing will result in pasty potatoes. Add ground black pepper to taste.

"One potato, two potato, three potato, four."
Child's rhyme

The refrigerator light goes on...
These potatoes have more butter in them than other Dr. Gourmet mashed potato recipes. This is to help enhance the creaminess and the mouthfeel that other flavors like roasted garlic or pesto achieve with less fat.

Nutrition Facts

Serving size	about 1 cup
Servings	4
Calories 119	Calories from Fat 21
	(% Daily Value)
Total Fat 2 g	(4 %)
Saturated Fat 2 g	(8 %)
Trans Fats 0 g	
Monounsaturated Fat 0 g	
Cholesterol 7 mg	(2 %)
Sodium 178 mg	(7 %)
Total Carbohydrates 21 g	(7 %)
Dietary Fiber 1 g	(10 %)
Sugars 2 g	
Protein 3 g	
Vitamin A 1 %	Vitamin C 38 %
Calcium 5 %	Iron 5 %
Vitamin K 2 mcg	
Potassium 532 mg	Magnesium 30 mg

Refried Black Beans

Servings = 4
Serving size = about 1 cup

This recipe can be easily multiplied or divided in 2.
This recipe makes good leftovers. Reheat gently.

1 tsp	olive oil
1 large	onion (minced)
2 15 ounce cans	no salt added black beans (drained and rinsed)
1 small	chipotle in adobo (minced)
4 cups	water
1/2 tsp	salt
1/2 tsp	cumin
to taste	fresh ground black pepper

Place the olive oil in a medium sauce pan over medium heat. Add the onion and cook for about 3 minutes.

Add the black beans, chipotle, water, salt, cumin and pepper. Stir well.

Simmer over medium heat stirring occasionally. Using a fork, spoon or potato masher, mash some of the black beans occasionally as they cook.

As the beans cook, add additional water if needed to keep the beans from getting too dried out. Stir and continue to mash the beans. After about 20 – 25 minutes the refried beans will begin to thicken up. Serve.

"If you are a dreamer, come in. If you are a dreamer, a wisher, a liar, a hoper, a prayer, a magic-bean-buyer. If you're a pretender, come sit by my fire, for we have some flax-golden tales to spin. Come in! Come in!"

Shel Silverstein, Poet

The refrigerator light goes on...
Refried beans aren't really refried. They are essentially simmered until the beans are well cooked and the carbohydrates help create a thick side dish. Often there's a lot of lard or other fat, but it's not really necessary for making a great dish of refried beans.

Nutrition Facts

| Serving size | about 1 cup |
| Servings | 4 |

Calories 196	Calories from Fat 17
	(% Daily Value)
Total Fat 2 g	(3 %)
Saturated Fat <1 g	(2 %)
Trans Fats 0 g	
Monounsaturated Fat 1 g	
Cholesterol 0 mg	(0 %)
Sodium 294 mg	(12 %)
Total Carbohydrates 34 g	(11 %)
Dietary Fiber 12 g	(48 %)
Sugars 2 g	
Protein 12 g	
Vitamin A 1 %	Vitamin C 7 %
Calcium 5 %	Iron 17 %
Vitamin K 1 mcg	
Potassium 521 mg	Magnesium 95 mg

Risotto with Peas

Servings = 2
Serving size = about 1 1/2 cups

This recipe will keep fairly well for about 48 hours in the fridge. Reheat gently.

1 tsp	grapeseed or extra virgin olive oil
1/2 large	onion
1/2 cup	arborio rice
1/4 tsp	salt
to taste	fresh ground black pepper
1 cup	low sodium chicken or vegetable broth
3 cups	water
2/3 cup	frozen peas
1 ounce	Parmigiano-Reggiano

Place the olive oil in the bottom of a large skillet. Heat over medium and add the onion. Cook gently, stirring frequently, until the onions just begin to turn translucent.

Add the arborio rice and stir. Cook for about 2 minutes and then add the salt and pepper. Add the chicken stock and enough water to cover the rice. Simmer on medium, partially covered for about 15 minutes. Check to see how close the rice is to being done and add more water if needed. The rice is done when it is still slightly firm but there is no grainy texture when chewed.

Add the peas and Parmigiano. Add a little more water if needed and cook for about 3 - 5 minutes until the peas are heated through.

"It suddenly struck me that that tiny pea, pretty and blue, was the Earth. I put up my thumb and shut one eye, and my thumb blotted out the planet Earth. I didn't feel like a giant. I felt very, very small."

Neil Armstrong, Astronaut

The refrigerator light goes on...
I have a lot of risotto dishes on the Dr. Gourmet Web site that are complete meals. I love to serve risotto with other main course recipes, however. This Risotto with Peas goes especially good with fish.

Of note, there's about 600 mg of sodium in this dish. While this is more than I generally like to use for side dishes, the recipe is both a starch *and* a veggie. Rice is just that way – it takes a little bit more salt to make the flavor pop and the recipe taste great.

Nutrition Facts

Serving size	about 1 1/2 cups
Servings	2

Calories 329	Calories from Fat 62
	(% Daily Value)
Total Fat 7 g	(11 %)
Saturated Fat 3 g	(14 %)
Trans Fats 0 g	
Monounsaturated Fat 2 g	
Cholesterol 10 mg	(3 %)
Sodium 606 mg	(25 %)
Total Carbohydrates 52 g	(17 %)
Dietary Fiber 1 g	(17 %)
Sugars 5 g	
Protein 14 g	
Vitamin A 20 %	Vitamin C 20 %
Calcium 19 %	Iron 18 %
Vitamin K 11 mcg	
Potassium 295 mg	Magnesium 35 mg

Roasted Acorn Squash

Servings = 2
Serving size = 1/2 squash

This recipe can be easily multiplied. The leftovers make a good ingredient in tossed salads.

1	acorn squash (about 1 pound)
1 tsp.	butter
2 tsp.	brown sugar

Preheat oven to 400°F.

Halve the squash lengthwise. Scoop out the seeds and discard them. Make shallow cuts in a grid pattern along the inside of the squash.

Place 1/2 teaspoon butter and 1/2 teaspoon brown sugar in the cavity of each squash.

Set the squash in the preheated oven and reduce the heat to 350°F. Roast for approximately 30 minutes. Using a spoon occasionally baste the top and inside of the squash with the sugar/butter mixture.

Remove and serve after allowing to cool for about 5 minutes.

"Many so-called aphrodisiac recipes are basically wholesome ingredients prepared in a tasty way. The receptivity to romance probably comes from the general sense of relaxation and well-being good food induces."

Harry E. Wedeck, Author,
The Dictionary of Pagan Religions

The refrigerator light goes on...
Simple dishes are the best. Pair this roasted acorn squash with a roasted salmon dish like the Salmon with Caper Mayonnaise and you have the nearly perfect meal.

Nutrition Facts

Serving size	1/2 squash
Servings	2
Calories 112	Calories from Fat 19
	(% Daily Value)
Total Fat 2 g	(3 %)
Saturated Fat 1 g	(6 %)
Trans Fats 0 g	
Monounsaturated Fat 1 g	
Cholesterol 5 mg	(2 %)
Sodium 8 mg	(0 %)
Total Carbohydrates 25 g	(8 %)
Dietary Fiber 3 g	(13 %)
Sugars 2 g	
Protein 2 g	
Vitamin A 17 %	Vitamin C 40 %
Calcium 7 %	Iron 9 %
Vitamin K 0 mcg	
Potassium 756 mg	Magnesium 70 mg

Roasted Beets

Servings = 4
Serving Size = about 1 cup

This recipe can easily be multiplied by 2, 3 or 4, but a larger roasting pan must be used. Leftovers are great ingredients in tossed salads.

2	medium beets
1 tsp.	unsalted butter
1/4 tsp.	salt
1/8 tsp.	dried oregano
1/8 tsp.	chili powder

Preheat the oven to 400°F.

Wrap the beets in a paper towel and cook on high in microwave for 5 minutes. Let cool for 5 minutes.

Peel and cut into 1 inch cubes.

Place in a roasting pan large enough so that the beets are not completely touching.

Put the pat of butter on the beets and sprinkle the salt, oregano and chili powder over the top.

Reduce the heat to 375°F and roast for 20 – 25 minutes. The beets are done when they are slightly crisp on the outside.

Chill at least 4 hours.

"The beet is the most intense of vegetables. The radish, admittedly, is more feverish, but the fire of the radish is a cold fire, the fire of discontent, not of passion. Tomatoes are lusty enough, yet there runs through tomatoes an undercurrent of frivolity. Beets are deadly serious."

Tom Robbins, Author

The refrigerator light goes on...
Roasting is an essential technique in cooking great healthy food. The most important thing is that the roasting pan be large enough so that the food doesn't touch. If you use too small a pan, the food will steam and not have that crispy outside the makes roasted food so great.

Nutrition Facts

Serving size	about 1 cup beets
Servings	4
Calories 44	Calories from Fat 10
	(% Daily Value)
Total Fat 1 g	(2 %)
Saturated Fat 1 g	(3 %)
Trans Fats 0 g	
Monounsaturated Fat 0 g	
Cholesterol 2 mg	(1 %)
Sodium 210 mg	(9 %)
Total Carbohydrates 8 g	(3 %)
Dietary Fiber 2 g	(9 %)
Sugars 6 g	
Protein 1 g	
Vitamin A 2 %	Vitamin C 7 %
Calcium 1 %	Iron 4 %
Vitamin K 0 mcg	
Potassium 269 mg	Magnesium 19 mg

Roasted Butternut Squash

Servings = 2
Serving size = about 1/2 squash

This recipe can easily be multiplied as many times as you have oven space for and makes great leftovers. Cut into chunks and serve cold in salads or reheat gently.

1 lb	butternut squash
	spray olive oil
2 tsp	unsalted butter
to taste	fresh ground black pepper
1/8 tsp	salt (divided)

Preheat oven to 375F.

Slice the squash lengthwise and scoop out the seeds.

Spray a skillet with the oil and place the squash in the pan face down, then place in the oven.

Bake for 30 minutes, then turn over and place 1 teaspoon butter, 1 teaspoon maple syrup and half the salt in the hollow of each squash. Grind the fresh pepper over the top and return to the oven, baking for another 15 minutes.

Serve.

"You know, when you get your first asparagus, or your first acorn squash, or your first really good tomato of the season, those are the moments that define the cook's year. I get more excited by that than anything else."

Mario Batali, Chef

The refrigerator light goes on...
There are a lot Dr. Gourmet recipes that use butternut squash (try the Butternut Squash Risotto). It has a sweet, nutty flavor similar to pumpkin. It is also similar to acorn squash in texture but usually sweeter. Choose smooth skinned butternut squash with no dark spots or blemishes. Both acorn and butternut squash are high in fiber: about 2 - 3 grams per cup of cubed squash.

Nutrition Facts

Serving size	about 1/2 squash
Servings	2
Calories 136	Calories from Fat 37
	(% Daily Value)
Total Fat 4 g	(6 %)
Saturated Fat 2 g	(10 %)
Trans Fat 0 g	
Monounsaturated Fat 1 g	
Cholesterol 10 mg	(3 %)
Sodium 155 mg	(6 %)
Total Carbohydrates 26 g	(8 %)
Dietary Fiber 5 g	(16 %)
Sugars 5 g	
Protein 2 g	
Vitamin A 466 %	Vitamin C 80 %
Calcium 8 %	Iron 8 %
Vitamin K 2 mcg	
Potassium 799 mg	Magnesium 77 mg

Roasted Corn on the Cob

Servings = 2
Serving size = 1 ear corn

This recipe can easily be multiplied as many times as you have room in the oven or grill for. I love leftover corn. Leave it wrapped in the husks inside the foil.

2	ears corn
1/8 tsp	pepper
1/4 tsp	salt
2 tsp	unsalted butter

Preheat the oven to 400°F.

Peel the husk back from the corn, being careful not to detach them from the stem. Remove silks and rinse well, wetting down the husks.

Sprinkle the salt and pepper over the corn.

Fold the husks against the corn and wrap in foil.

Roast in the oven for about 30 minutes. Turn them 1/4 turn about every 7 – 8 minutes.

Remove from the oven and unwrap the foil. Cut the bottom of the cob so that the husks fall away easily.

Serve each with a pat of butter.

These can also be roasted on top of the grill. The heat should be medium to medium-high and you must turn them frequently, as noted above.

"The greatest drawback is the way in which it is necessary to eat it. It looks awkward enough: but what is to be done? Surrendering such a vegetable from considerations of grace is not to be thought of."

Harriet Martineau, an Englishwoman writing about corn on the cob in 1835

The refrigerator light goes on...
This recipe includes the pat of butter for your corn on the cob because it just wouldn't be corn without it. Take the pat and enjoy it. This recipe works well both on the grill and in the oven. The grill will give the corn a lovely charcoal flavor.

Nutrition Facts

Serving size	1 ear corn
Servings	2
Calories 144	Calories from Fat 44
	(% Daily Value)
Total Fat 5 g	(8 %)
Saturated Fat 3 g	(13 %)
Trans Fat 0 g	
Monounsaturated Fat 1 g	
Cholesterol 10 mg	(3 %)
Sodium 320 mg	(13 %)
Total Carbohydrates 26 g	(9 %)
Dietary Fiber 3 g	(11 %)
Sugars 4 g	
Protein 3 g	
Vitamin A 2 %	Vitamin C 11 %
Calcium 0 %	Iron 4 %
Vitamin K 1 mcg	
Potassium 258 mg	Magnesium 33 mg

Roasted Garlic

Servings = 6
Serving size = 1/3 head of garlic (about 6 cloves)

I make up to about 4 heads of garlic at a time. This keeps well, tightly covered, for about 4 - 6 days.

2	heads whole garlic
2 tsp	extra virgin olive oil

Preheat oven to 300°F.

Peel the outermost skin of the garlic only. With the bulb whole, turn on its side and slice 1/2-inch of the stem end off the garlic bulbs.

Pour the olive oil in the bottom of a heavy bottom sauce pan.

Place the garlic cut side down in the pan.

Cover and roast for 45 minutes until cloves are slightly brown at the cut end and soft throughout.

"There is no such thing as a little garlic."
Arthur Baer, Investment Author

The refrigerator light goes on...
Roasted garlic is a staple in my kitchen and should be in yours. I generally roast about 3 heads every ten days or so. It makes a great ingredient in mashed potatoes and also enriches any sauce. It is fantastic served as hors d'oeuvres on bread with some soft goat cheese and veggies.

Nutrition Facts

Serving size	1/3 head of garlic (about 6 cloves)
Servings	6
Calories 40	Calories from Fat 14
	(% Daily Value)
Total Fat 2 g	(2 %)
Saturated Fat 0 g	(1 %)
Trans Fat 0 g	
Monounsaturated Fat 0 g	
Cholesterol 0 mg	(0 %)
Sodium 3 mg	(0 %)
Total Carbohydrates 6 g	(2 %)
Dietary Fiber 0 g	(2 %)
Sugars 0 g	
Protein 1 g	
Vitamin A 0 %	Vitamin C 9 %
Calcium 3 %	Iron 2 %
Vitamin K 1 mcg	
Potassium 72 mg	Magnesium 5 mg

Roasted Garlic Mashed Potatoes

Servings = 4
Serving size = about 1 cup

This recipe can easily be multiplied. These do not keep very well. This recipe requires Roasted Garlic to be made first (recipe included).

3 quarts	water
1 lb	Yukon Gold potatoes
2 tsp	unsalted butter
1/3 cup	non-fat buttermilk
1/3 cup	2% milk
1/2 tsp	salt
4 cloves	roasted garlic

Place the water in a large stock-pot over high heat.

Quarter the potatoes and add them to the stock-pot. Cover with water by about an inch. Bring to boil and then reduce heat until the water is simmering.

Cook the potatoes about 15 – 20 minutes, until slightly soft in the middle. They should give when squeezed.

Remove from heat and drain water. Add butter, buttermilk, milk, salt and roasted garlic. Mash potatoes until creamy and the roasted garlic is well blended. I like to leave some chunks of potatoes. If you like them smooth, be careful because over mashing will result in pasty potatoes.

Add ground black pepper to taste.

"I have made a lot of mistakes falling in love, and regretted most of them, but never the potatoes that went with them."

Nora Ephron, Screenwriter

The refrigerator light goes on...
The key to good mashed potatoes is in the buttermilk / milk combination. The buttermilk adds richness and tartness, with no fat and the milk adds creaminess. The butter is used here only as a flavor enhancer.

Nutrition Facts

Serving size	about 1 cup
Servings	4
Calories 130	Calories from Fat 24
	(% Daily Value)
Total Fat 3 g	(4 %)
Saturated Fat 2 g	(6 %)
Trans Fat 0 g	
Monounsaturated Fat 1 g	
Cholesterol 7 mg	(2 %)
Sodium 176 mg	(7 %)
Total Carbohydrates 23 g	(8 %)
Dietary Fiber 3 g	(10 %)
Sugars 3 g	
Protein 4 g	
Vitamin A 2 %	Vitamin C 40 %
Calcium 7 %	Iron 5 %
Vitamin K 3 mcg	
Potassium 564 mg	Magnesium 33 mg

Roasted Garlic Succotash

Servings = 2
Serving size = about 1 cup

This recipe can be multiplied as many times as you like. This recipe requires Roasted Garlic to be made first (recipe included).

1	ear corn (cut kernels from cob)
1/2 cup	water
1/8 tsp	salt
to taste	fresh ground black pepper
1 cup	frozen lima beans
4 cloves	roasted garlic
1 tsp	unsalted butter

Place the corn kernels and water in a small sauce pan over medium high heat. Bring the water to a boil and immediately reduce the heat until the corn is simmering.

Add the salt and pepper. Cook for about 7 – 10 minutes until the water is almost evaporated.

Add the lima beans and cook for about 3 minutes until the water has almost evaporated.

Mash the roasted garlic into the butter using the tines of a fork. Place the garlic butter in the pan and toss until melted. Serve.

"Charlie Sheen, Ben Vereen, shrink to the size of a lima bean."

Brain (of Pinky and the Brain)

The refrigerator light goes on...
Adding roasted garlic makes a rich and creamy succotash. Another good reason to keep roasted garlic on hand.

Nutrition Facts

Serving size	about 1 cup
Servings	2
Calories 201	Calories from Fat 32
	(% Daily Value)
Total Fat 4 g	(6 %)
Saturated Fat 1 g	(7 %)
Trans Fat 0 g	
Monounsaturated Fat 1 g	
Cholesterol 4 mg	(2 %)
Sodium 173 mg	(7 %)
Total Carbohydrates 37 g	(12 %)
Dietary Fiber 7 g	(27 %)
Sugars 4 g	
Protein 9 g	
Vitamin A 6 %	Vitamin C 26 %
Calcium 4 %	Iron 14 %
Vitamin K 6 mcg	
Potassium 717 mg	Magnesium 93 mg

Roasted Parsnips and Carrots

Servings = 4
Serving size = about 4 ounces veggies

This recipe can be multiplied (or divided by 2) but will need multiple pans. Keeps well, refrigerated, for 3-4 days. Great hot or cold.

8 ounces	carrots (peeled and sliced into rounds)
8 ounces	parsnips (peeled and sliced into rounds)
1 Tbsp	olive oil
1/2 tsp	dried thyme
1/4 tsp	salt
to taste	fresh ground black pepper

Place a stainless steel skillet in the oven and preheat the oven to 425F.

Fold the carrots, parsnips, thyme, salt, and pepper together and place in the preheated skillet and return to the oven.

Reduce the oven heat to 375F.

Roast the carrots and parsnips for about 25 minutes, stirring once or twice, until the carrots and parsnips are softened.

Serve hot or allow to cool in a non-reactive bowl, then refrigerate.

"The day is coming when a single carrot, freshly observed, will set off a revolution."
Paul Cezanne, Artist

The refrigerator light goes on...
While this recipe is cooking your house will fill up with the lovely aroma of thyme. Great hot or cold, take this dish to your next potluck: easy, colorful and delicious.

Nutrition Facts

Serving size	about 4 ounces veggies
Servings	4
Calories 96	Calories from Fat 33
	(% Daily Value)
Total Fat 3 g	(5 %)
Saturated Fat 0 g	(2 %)
Trans Fat 0 g	
Monounsaturated Fat 2 g	
Cholesterol 0 mg	(0 %)
Sodium 190 mg	(8 %)
Total Carbohydrates 15 g	(6 %)
Dietary Fiber 5 g	(16 %)
Sugars 6 g	
Protein 2 g	
Vitamin A 182 %	Vitamin C 22 %
Calcium 4 %	Iron 3 %
Vitamin K 24 mcg	
Potassium 395 mg	Magnesium 23 mg

Roasted Potatoes

Servings = 4
Serving size = about 1 cup

This recipe can be multiplied but does not keep well.

3 quarts	water
1 lb	medium red or Yukon gold potatoes
2 tsp	unsalted butter
1 cloves	garlic
1 Tbsp	fresh parsley
1 Tbsp	fresh chives
1/4 tsp	salt
1/8 tsp	chili powder

Preheat oven to 400° F.

Place the water in a medium stock pot over high heat and bring to a boil. Add the potatoes and reduce the heat to medium-high. Simmer for 10 minutes and remove. Drain potatoes and let them cool slightly before cutting them into quarters.

Place potatoes in a roasting pan large enough so that they are not crowded.

Put the butter on top and sprinkle the garlic, parsley, chives, salt and chili powder over the potatoes.

Place the pan in the oven and roast for about 25 –30 minutes. As soon as the butter has melted stir the potatoes and then stir them gently about every five minutes.

They are done when they are slightly crisp on the outside (about 20 – 25 minutes).

"If the divine creator has taken pains to give us delicious and exquisite things to eat, the least we can do is prepare them well and serve them with ceremony."

Fernand Point, 20th century French chef

The refrigerator light goes on...
If you are in a hurry wrap the potatoes in a paper towel and cook on high in microwave for 3 minutes instead of boiling them.

Nutrition Facts

Serving size	about 1 cup
Servings	4
Calories 106	Calories from Fat 18
	(% Daily Value)
Total Fat 2 g	(3 %)
Saturated Fat 1 g	(6 %)
Trans Fat 0 g	
Monounsaturated Fat 0 g	
Cholesterol 5 mg	(2 %)
Sodium 153 mg	(6 %)
Total Carbohydrates 20 g	(7 %)
Dietary Fiber 3 g	(10 %)
Sugars 1 g	
Protein 2 g	
Vitamin A 3 %	Vitamin C 41 %
Calcium 2 %	Iron 5 %
Vitamin K 19 mcg	
Potassium 591 mg	Magnesium 27 mg

Roasted Tomatoes

Servings = 2
Serving size = 2 tomatoes

This recipe can easily be multiplied but does not keep well past one day.

	spray olive oil
4 medium	tomatoes
1/8 tsp.	salt
to taste	fresh ground black pepper

Preheat the oven to 375°F. Place a large skillet in the oven.

When the oven is hot lightly spray the pan with olive oil and place the tomatoes in stem side down.

Roast for 30 minutes and remove from the oven. Turn the tomatoes over so they are stem side up resting in the hot pan and let them cool in the pan for 30 minutes.

Chill.

After they are cold, using a very sharp paring knife, gently cut the stem and core from the tomato.

"My greatest strength is... common sense. I'm really a standard brand like Campbell's tomato soup or Baker's chocolate."
Katharine Hepburn, Actress

The refrigerator light goes on...
You could sprinkle about 1/8 tsp salt over these after cooking, but I like the simple sweetness of the roasted tomatoes, especially when I am going to use them as an accompaniment for a salad or other dish that might be tart or salty.

Nutrition Facts

Serving size	2 tomatoes
Servings	2
Calories 44	Calories from Fat 4
	(% Daily Value)
Total Fat 0 g	(1 %)
Saturated Fat 0 g	(0 %)
Trans Fat 0 g	
Monounsaturated Fat 0 g	
Cholesterol 0 mg	(0 %)
Sodium 158 mg	(7 %)
Total Carbohydrates 10 g	(3 %)
Dietary Fiber 3 g	(12 %)
Sugars 6 g	
Protein 2 g	
Vitamin A 41 %	Vitamin C 52 %
Calcium 2 %	Iron 4 %
Vitamin K 19 mcg	
Potassium 583 mg	Magnesium 27 mg

Roasted Vegetables with Caper Vinaigrette

Servings = 4
Serving size = about 1 1/2 cups

This recipe can easily be multiplied. This recipe makes great leftovers and is good served hot or cold.

1 quart	water
8 ounces	green beans
1 large	eggplant (sliced into 1/8ths lengthwise)
	spray olive oil
1 small	red onion (sliced into 1/8ths lengthwise)
1 large	red bell pepper (seeded and sliced into 1/8ths lengthwise
1 large	green bell pepper (seeded and sliced into 1/8ths lengthwise)
2 Tbsp.	olive oil
1 Tbsp.	balsamic vinegar
2 tsp.	coarse ground mustard
1 Tbsp.	maple syrup
1/8 tsp.	salt
to taste	fresh ground black pepper
4 tsp.	capers

Preheat the oven to 325°F.

Place the water in a medium pot over high heat. When the water begins to boil reduce the heat to keep it at barely a simmer.

Add the green beans and blanch for 3 minutes. Remove to a paper towel.

Place the eggplant on a cookie sheet and spray with olive oil. Place the eggplant in the oven.

Place the peppers, onions and green beans on a separate cookie sheet, spray lightly with olive oil and place in the oven.

Roast the eggplant, turning twice, for about 25 minutes. Stir the veggies on the other cookie sheet during roasting.

While the vegetables are roasting place the olive oil, vinegar, mustard, maple syrup, salt and pepper in a large mixing bowl. Whisk until smooth.

When the veggies are soft (but not too limp) remove from the oven. Place the peppers, onions and green beans in the bowl with the vinaigrette.

Let the eggplant cool for a couple of minutes and cut crosswise into 1 inch pieces. Add to the bowl.

Toss the veggies to coat with the dressing.

Add the capers and toss. Serve.

"I think of New York as a puree and the rest of the United States as vegetable soup."
Spalding Gray, Essayist

The refrigerator light goes on...
You can use almost any vegetable for this recipe. The key is to choose those that are softer and will roast in about 20 to 25 minutes. Zucchini or yellow squash would work, as will mushrooms. If you are going to include firmer choices, like carrots or parsnips, blanch them for a few minutes along with the green beans to precook them prior to roasting.

Nutrition Facts

Serving size	about 1 1/2 cups
Servings	4

Calories 160	Calories from Fat 67
	(% Daily Value)
Total Fat 7 g	(11 %)
Saturated Fat 1 g	(4 %)
Trans Fat 0 g	
Monounsaturated Fat 5 g	
Cholesterol 0 mg	(0 %)
Sodium 196 mg	(8 %)
Total Carbohydrates 21 g	(10 %)
Dietary Fiber 9 g	(26 %)
Sugars 12 g	
Protein 2 g	
Vitamin A 42 %	Vitamin C 167 %
Calcium 4 %	Iron 6 %
Vitamin K 22 mcg	
Potassium 619 mg	Magnesium 48 mg

Rosemary Potatoes

Servings = 2
Serving size = about 1 cup

This recipe can easily be multiplied. Leftovers are fair - reheated potatoes will not be as crispy.

3 quarts	water
12 ounces	medium red or Yukon Gold potatoes
1 tsp	unsalted butter
1 tsp	olive oil
1 clove	garlic (minced)
2 tsp	dried rosemary
1/8 tsp	salt
to taste	fresh ground black pepper

Preheat oven to 325° F.

Place the water in a medium stock pot over high heat and bring to a boil. Add the potatoes and reduce the heat to medium-high. Simmer for 10 minutes and remove. Drain potatoes and let them cool slightly before cutting them into quarters.

Place potatoes in a roasting pan large enough so that they are not crowded.

Put the butter and olive oil on top and sprinkle the garlic, rosemary, salt and pepper over the potatoes.

Place the pan in the oven and roast for about 25 –30 minutes. As soon as the butter has melted stir the potatoes and then stir them gently about every five minutes.

They are done when they are slightly crisp on the outside (about 20 – 25 minutes).

"Without the potato, the balance of European power might never have tilted north."
Michael Pollan, Author

The refrigerator light goes on...
Rosemary and potatoes are just made for each other. This is a quick and easy fresh recipe. If you're really in a hurry, place the potatoes in the microwave for 1 minute on high. Turn them and then microwave on high for a second minute. Remove and let cool for a minute or so. Cut into chunks and then proceed with the third step, putting the potatoes in the roasting pan with the other ingredients.

Nutrition Facts

Serving size	about 1 cup
Servings	2
Calories 171	Calories from Fat 39
	(% Daily Value)
Total Fat 4 g	(7 %)
Saturated Fat 2 g	(8 %)
Trans Fat 0 g	
Monounsaturated Fat 2 g	
Cholesterol 5 mg	(2 %)
Sodium 156 mg	(7 %)
Total Carbohydrates 32 g	(11 %)
Dietary Fiber 4 g	(17 %)
Sugars 1 g	
Protein 4 g	
Vitamin A 2 %	Vitamin C 57 %
Calcium 4 %	Iron 9 %
Vitamin K 5 mcg	
Potassium 724 mg	Magnesium 1 mg

Southern Green Beans

Servings = 4
Serving size = about 1 1/2 cups beans

This recipe can easily be multiplied.

2 slices	bacon (diced)
1 small	onion (diced)
1 lb.	green beans (trimmed & cut into 1 1/2 inch pieces)
1/2 tsp.	sugar
1/4 tsp.	salt
to taste	fresh ground black pepper

Place a large sauce pan over high heat. Add the diced bacon and cook, stirring frequently, for about 5 minutes. Reduce the heat if needed so that the bacon doesn't burn.

Add the onions and cook for about 2 minutes.

Add the green beans, sugar, salt, and pepper. Stir and cover.

Reduce the heat to medium low and cook for about 30 minutes, stirring occasionally.

"I like health-conscious cooking, but growing up in the South, I do love southern cooking; southern France, southern Italy, southern Spain. I love southern cooking."

Clarence Clemons, Musician

The refrigerator light goes on...
You can cook these as long as you want. True Southern beans are cooked to heck and gone and I do love them that way.

Nutrition Facts

Serving size	about 1 1/2 cups beans
Servings	4
Calories 115	Calories from Fat 62
	(% Daily Value)
Total Fat 7 g	(11 %)
Saturated Fat 2 g	(11 %)
Trans Fat 0 g	
Monounsaturated Fat 3 g	
Cholesterol 10 mg	(3 %)
Sodium 278 mg	(12 %)
Total Carbohydrates 11 g	(4 %)
Dietary Fiber 4 g	(17 %)
Sugars 3 g	
Protein 4 g	
Vitamin A 16 %	Vitamin C 33 %
Calcium 5 %	Iron 7 %
Vitamin K 16 mcg	
Potassium 301 mg	Magnesium 32 mg

Southwest Succotash

Servings = 2
Serving size = about 1 cup

This recipe can easily be multiplied as many times as you like. Leftovers are fair.

1 tsp	olive oil
1 medium	green onion (sliced crosswise)
1	ear corn (kernels cut from cob)
1 cup	frozen lima beans
1/8 tsp	salt
to taste	fresh ground black pepper
1/8 tsp	ground cumin
1/8 tsp	chili powder
1/4 tsp	paprika
1/2 cup	water

Place the olive oil in a medium skillet over medium high heat. Add the green onion and cook for about 30 seconds stirring constantly.

Add the corn kernels. Cook, tossing, frequently, for about 10 minutes. If the corn begins to brown too fast, reduce the heat.

Add the lima beans, salt, pepper, cumin, chili powder, and paprika. Toss for about minute.

Add the water and cook for about 4 – 5 minutes until the water is almost evaporated. Serve.

"A light wind swept over the corn, and all nature laughed in the sunshine."

Anne Bronte, Author

The refrigerator light goes on...
My mom served Succotash when I was a kid, but it was frozen. I like it still, but this is a great riff on the corn and lima combo. This Southwest Succotash is not too spicy and if you want to zip it up, add a bit of cayenne pepper.

Nutrition Facts

Serving size	about 1 cup
Servings	2
Calories 195	Calories from Fat 31
	(% Daily Value)
Total Fat 4 g	(5 %)
Saturated Fat 1 g	(3 %)
Trans Fat 0 g	
Monounsaturated Fat 2 g	
Cholesterol 0 mg	(0 %)
Sodium 174 mg	(7 %)
Total Carbohydrates 36 g	(12 %)
Dietary Fiber 7 g	(28 %)
Sugars 4 g	
Protein 8 g	
Vitamin A 10 %	Vitamin C 26 %
Calcium 4 %	Iron 26 %
Vitamin K 6 mcg	
Potassium 724 mg	Magnesium 23 mg

Steamed Artichoke

Servings = 1
Serving size = 1 medium artichoke

This recipe can easily be multiplied as many times as you like. This recipe keeps well in the refrigerator for 48 hours.

| 1 quart | water |
| 1 medium | artichoke |

Place the water in a medium pan fitted with a steamer basket over high heat.

Using scissors clip about 1/4 inch off of the tip of the artichoke leaves. Trim the stem to the base of the artichoke.

Place the artichoke in the steamer and reduce the heat until the water is simmering. Cover.

Steam for 25 minutes. Turn off the heat and let stand for 5 minutes.

Serve warm or cold with dipping sauce.

"Life is like eating artichokes, you have got to go through so much to get so little."
Thomas Aloysius Dorgan, Cartoonist

The refrigerator light goes on...
Artichokes make the perfect dinner party appetizer. They're easy to prepare, keep well overnight and you can pair them with almost any dipping sauce you like. While the traditional dip is drawn butter, any of your favorite dressings or sauces will do. Try Blue Cheese dressing or even Sauce Romesco. Using a vinaigrette will be especially healthy, and flavored olive oils like truffle oil or basil oil work great.

Nutrition Facts

Serving size	1 medium artichoke
Servings	1
Calories 64	Calories from Fat 3
	(% Daily Value)
Total Fat 0 g	(1 %)
Saturated Fat 0 g	(0 %)
Trans Fat 0 g	
Monounsaturated Fat 0 g	
Cholesterol 0 mg	(0 %)
Sodium 72 mg	(3 %)
Total Carbohydrates 14 g	(5 %)
Dietary Fiber 10 g	(41 %)
Sugars 1 g	
Protein 3 g	
Vitamin A 0 %	Vitamin C 15 %
Calcium 3 %	Iron 4 %
Vitamin K 18 mcg	
Potassium 343 mg	Magnesium 50 mg

Sweet Potato and Poblano Home Fries

Servings = 2
Serving size = about 1 cup

This recipe can easily be multiplied as many times as you like. Leftovers are pretty good. Reheat gently.

1 medium	poblano pepper
1 tsp	olive oil
1 medium	red onion (diced)
8 ounces	sweet potatoes (yams) (1/2 inch dice)
1/2 tsp	paprika
1/4 tsp	cumin
1/4 tsp	salt
to taste	fresh ground black pepper

Preheat the oven to 325°F.

Place the pepper in the oven and roast, about 30 minutes, until the outside is charred.

Place the roasted pepper in a paper bag and fold over the top, then allow to cool for ten minutes. After ten minutes, the roasted skin should slip off easily. Seed the peeled poblano and dice.

Place the olive oil in a medium saucepan over medium-high heat. Add the onions and cook until they begin to caramelize, about 7-10 minutes.

Add the diced yams, toss well, and cover. Cook for about ten minutes over medium-high heat, stirring occasionally, until the yams are slightly tender.

Add the poblano peppers, the paprika, cumin, salt and pepper and stir. Recover and allow to cook for another 5-10 minutes, stirring occasionally, until the yams are soft.

Serve.

"He that but looketh on a plate of ham and eggs to lust after it hath already committed breakfast with it in his heart."

C.S. Lewis

The refrigerator light goes on...
This is a fairly spicy recipe, so if you like your food a little milder, substitute half a roasted green bell pepper for half of the poblano pepper.

The key to making home fries like those you get at a restaurant is to use a little bit of oil and a moderately hot pan. After caramelizing the onions and adding the potatoes I reduce the heat slightly and cover. The steam helps increase the heat and cook the potatoes through. If you stir only about every three minutes, the bottom layer of the potatoes will brown nicely but not stick to the pan. Toss them, pat down slightly cover and repeat. Keep a close watch on this dish in the last ten minutes or so of cooking, as you want the onions, peppers and sweet potatoes to caramelize, but not burn.

Nutrition Facts

Serving size	about 1 cup
Servings	1

Calories 191	Calories from Fat 25
	(% Daily Value)
Total Fat 2 g	(4 %)
Saturated Fat 0 g	(1 %)
Trans Fat 0 g	
Monounsaturated Fat 2 g	
Cholesterol 0 mg	(0 %)
Sodium 305 mg	(12 %)
Total Carbohydrates 4 g	(15 %)
Dietary Fiber 7 g.	(24 %)
Sugars 4 g	
Protein 4 g	
Vitamin A 13 %	Vitamin C 120 %
Calcium 3 %	Iron 8 %
Vitamin K 8 mcg	
Potassium 1126 mg	Magnesium 38 mg

Thick Cut Yam Home Fries

Servings = 2
Serving size = about 1 1/2 cups fries

This recipe can easily be multiplied as many times as you like but does not make very good leftovers.

2 small	yams (about 5 ounces each)
1/4 tsp	salt
to taste	fresh ground black pepper
1/8 tsp	dried thyme leaves
	spray olive oil

Place a large skillet in the oven and set the preheat to 325°F.

Scrub the yams well and then cut into wedges. It's easiest to cut them in half lengthwise and then quarters and then eighths.

When the oven is hot spray the pan lightly with oil. Add the yam wedges and sprinkle the salt, pepper and thyme over the top. Spray lightly with olive oil.

Return the pan to the oven and cook for about 25 minutes, tossing frequently.

Serve hot.

"If life were fair, Dan Quayle would be making a living asking 'Do you want fries with that?'"
John Cleese, Genius

The refrigerator light goes on...
This recipe is so simple you just have to do it. The prep takes all of two minutes. Tossing them into a pan and watching them - another two minutes. Great fries to go with that burger in thirty minutes total. Easy!

Nutrition Facts

Serving size	about 1 1/2 cups fries
Servings	2
Calories 185	Calories from Fat 22
	(% Daily Value)
Total Fat 2 g	(4 %)
Saturated Fat 0 g	(2 %)
Trans Fat 0 g	
Monounsaturated Fat 2 g	
Cholesterol 0 mg	(0 %)
Sodium 303 mg	(13 %)
Total Carbohydrates 39 g	(13 %)
Dietary Fiber 6 g	(23 %)
Sugars 1 g	
Protein 2 g	
Vitamin A 4 %	Vitamin C 40 %
Calcium 3 %	Iron 5 %
Vitamin K 6 mcg	
Potassium 1143 mg	Magnesium 30 mg

Tomato Sauce

Servings = 10
Serving size = 1/2 cup

Keeps well in the fridge for about 4 – 5 days. Can also be frozen - try freezing single portions in plastic bags for those last-minute meals.

1 Tbsp	olive oil
6 cloves	garlic (minced)
1 small	onion (diced)
2 28 oz. cans	no salt added peeled tomatoes (chopped)
3 cups	water
1/4 tsp	salt

Place the oil in a large skillet and heat over a medium-high heat. Reduce the heat to medium and add the garlic. Cook gently for about 3 minutes. Do not allow the garlic to turn brown.

Add the onions and cook until they are translucent. Stir frequently and do not allow them to brown.

Add the tomatoes and water and reduce the heat to low. Cook until the tomatoes are soft (about 90 minutes).

Remove from heat, add the salt and puree until smooth with a stick or conventional blender.

"There is no love sincerer than the love of food."
George Bernard Shaw, Playwright

The refrigerator light goes on...
This recipe is based on using no salt added tomatoes. Having a low sodium (salt) sauce lets you add salt when using the sauce in other recipes.

Nutrition Facts

Serving size	1/2 cup
Servings	10
Calories 43	Calories from Fat 14
	(% Daily Value)
Total Fat 2 g	(2 %)
Saturated Fat 0 g	(1 %)
Trans Fat 0 g	
Monounsaturated Fat 0 g	
Cholesterol 0 mg	(0 %)
Sodium 21 mg	(1 %)
Total Carbohydrates 7 g	(2 %)
Dietary Fiber 2 g	(7 %)
Sugars 4 g	
Protein 1 g	
Vitamin A 4 %	Vitamin C 26 %
Calcium 5 %	Iron 9 %
Vitamin K 5 mcg	
Potassium 311 mg	Magnesium 18 mg

Warm Potato Salad

Servings = 6
Serving size = about 1 1/2 cups

This recipe can easily be multiplied. This recipe makes great leftovers. Reheat gently. This is also good served as cold potato salad.

4 quarts	water
2 lb	Yukon Gold or red potatoes (cut into 1 1/2 inch cubes)
3 Tbsp	olive oil
2 Tbsp	capers
2 Tbsp	caper juice
3	ribs celery (diced)
1/2 tsp	salt
to taste	fresh ground black pepper
1 tsp	fresh thyme leaves

Place the water in a large stock pot over high heat.

Add the potatoes to the stock pot. Bring to boil and then reduce heat until the water is at a slow boil.

Cook the potatoes about 10 - 15 minutes until slightly soft in the middle. They should be firm when squeezed.

Remove from heat and drain water.

Add the olive oil, capers, caper juice, celery, salt, pepper and thyme leaves. Toss well. Serve warm.

"Kissing a man with a beard is a lot like going to a picnic. You don't mind going through a little bush to get there!"

Minnie Pearl, Comedian

The refrigerator light goes on...
Warm potato salads are perfect for serving with a casual dinner party. A grilled steak, barbecue chicken or shrimp all make the perfect meal. The flavor of the olive oil, thyme and capers come through in the warm vinaigrette.

Nutrition Facts

Serving size	about 1 1/2 cups
Servings	6
Calories 181	Calories from Fat 62
	(% Daily Value)
Total Fat 7 g	(33 %)
Saturated Fat 1 g	(5 %)
Trans Fat 0 g	
Monounsaturated Fat 5 g	
Cholesterol 0 mg	(14 %)
Sodium 313 mg	(13 %)
Total Carbohydrates 29 g	(10 %)
Dietary Fiber 4 g	(16 %)
Sugars 2 g	
Protein 3 g	
Vitamin A 3 %	Vitamin C 51 %
Calcium 3 %	Iron 8 %
Vitamin K 18 mcg	
Potassium 714 mg	Magnesium 39 mg

Yam Home Fries

Servings = 4
Serving size = about 1 cup

This recipe can be multiplied but does not make very good leftovers.

2 Tbsp	light spread (like Promise Buttery Spread Light or Smart Balance Light)
1 large	shallot (diced)
1 lb	yams (diced)
1/4 tsp	salt
to taste	fresh ground black pepper
1/4 tsp	dried thyme leaves
1/4 tsp	dried oregano leaves

Place a large skillet in the oven and preheat oven to 325°F.

When the pan is hot add the spread, shallot and yams. Return the pan to the oven and cook for about ten minutes. Stir the yams and continue to roast in the oven stirring every 8 - 10 minutes. It will take about 30 minutes until the yams begin to soften.

Add the salt pepper, thyme and oregano and stir. Cook for another 5 - 8 minutes until the yams are slightly crispy on the outside and soft on the inside.

"To eat well in England you should have breakfast three times a day."

W. Somerset Maugham, Author

The refrigerator light goes on...
Yams make a great alternative to potatoes. They have pretty much the same texture but so much more character. Dishes like this will make your main course or breakfast shine. Best of all, they're really great for you.

Nutrition Facts

Serving size	about 1 cup
Servings	4

Calories 163	Calories from Fat 25
	(% Daily Value)
Total Fat 3 g	(4 %)
Saturated Fat 1 g	(4 %)
Trans Fat 0 g	
Monounsaturated Fat 1 g	
Cholesterol 0 mg	(0 %)
Sodium 201 mg	(8 %)
Total Carbohydrates 33 g	(11 %)
Dietary Fiber 5 g	(19 %)
Sugars 1 g	
Protein 2 g	
Vitamin A 12 %	Vitamin C 33 %
Calcium 2 %	Iron 4 %
Vitamin K 6 mcg	
Potassium 957 mg	Magnesium 26 mg

Yellow Squash and Onions

Servings = 2
Serving size = about 1 1/2 cups

This recipe can easily be multiplied but does not make very good leftovers.

1 tsp.	olive oil
1/2 small	white onion (sliced)
16 ounces	yellow squash (1/2 inch slices)
1/8 tsp.	salt
to taste	fresh ground black pepper

Place the olive oil in a large skillet over medium-high heat. Add the onion and cook for about 3 minutes until it begins to soften.

Add the yellow squash and cook, tossing frequently, for about 7 - 10 minutes. Cook the squash only until it just begins to soften, then add the salt and pepper.

Toss for one minute more and serve.

"Human beings, vegetables, or comic dust, we all dance to a mysterious tune, intoned in the distance by an invisible player,"
Albert Einstein, Physicist

The refrigerator light goes on...
I have loved yellow squash since I was a kid. Strange, I know, but my mother cooked great squash. The Southern tradition was to cook it much longer, but I like squash that's not as over-cooked as most people remember it. This recipe is quick and easy, full of flavor, and by not over-cooking the squash it has great texture.

Nutrition Facts

Serving size	about 1 1/2 cups
Servings	2
Calories 72	Calories from Fat 25
	(% Daily Value)
Total Fat 3 g	(4 %)
Saturated Fat 0 g	(2 %)
Trans Fat 0 g	
Monounsaturated Fat 2 g	
Cholesterol 0 mg	(14 %)
Sodium 157 mg	(7 %)
Total Carbohydrates 11 g	(4 %)
Dietary Fiber 5 g	(19 %)
Sugars 1 g	
Protein 2 g	
Vitamin A 7 %	Vitamin C 34 %
Calcium 5 %	Iron 6 %
Vitamin K 2 mcg	
Potassium 511 mg	Magnesium 50 mg

Yellow Squash with Red Peppers

Servings = 2
Serving size = about 1 1/2 cups

This recipe can be multiplied and makes great left-overs, in both salads and sandwiches.

1 tsp	olive oil
1/2 small	onion (diced)
1/2 medium	red bell pepper (diced)
2 large	yellow squash (about 1/2 pound each) (cut into 1/2 inch dice)
1/4 cup	water
1 tsp	dried oregano
1/8 tsp	salt
to taste	fresh ground black pepper

Place the olive oil in a medium skillet over medium high heat.

Add the onion and cook for about 2 minutes. Stir frequently.

Add the diced pepper and cook for about 2 minutes. Stir frequently.

Add the yellow squash and toss well.

Add the water, oregano, salt and pepper.

Cover and cook for about 15 minutes. Adjust the heat so that the squash doesn't cook too fast and risk burning.

When the squash is slightly tender remove the cover and cook for another two minutes. Serve.

"Bad cooks - and the utter lack of reason in the kitchen - have delayed human development longest and impaired it most."

Louis Diat, Chef

The refrigerator light goes on...
There is a balance between having squash that still has texture and squash that is soggy. The water helps the squash to steam but it isn't so much that they will get soggy. At the end of the cooking, increasing the heat to medium-high will help evaporate any extra liquid.

Sweet squash with onions and peppers only made better by the herbaceous oregano.

Nutrition Facts

Serving size	about 1 1/2 cups
Servings	2
Calories 88	Calories from Fat 26
	(% Daily Value)
Total Fat 3 g	(4 %)
Saturated Fat <1 g	(1 %)
Trans Fat 0 g	
Monounsaturated Fat 2 g	
Cholesterol 0 mg	(0 %)
Sodium 298 mg	(12 %)
Total Carbohydrates 14 g	(2 %)
Dietary Fiber 6 g	(21 %)
Sugars 2 g	
Protein 2 g	
Vitamin A 27 %	Vitamin C 101 %
Calcium 10 %	Iron 11 %
Vitamin K 5 mcg	
Potassium 603 mg	Magnesium 57 mg

Zucchini Pico de Gallo

Servings = 4
Serving size = about 1 cup

This recipe can easily be multiplied. This recipe
makes very good leftovers.

1 quart	water
4 medium	zucchini (about 1 pound) (cut into small dice)
1 small	shallot (finely minced)
1 large	tomato (diced)
1	lime (juiced)
1 Tbsp.	olive oil
1 tsp.	maple syrup
1/4 tsp.	salt
to taste	fresh ground black pepper
1/8 tsp.	red pepper flakes
1/2 tsp.	chili powder
1/2 cup	cilantro (chopped)

Place the water in a large stock pot over high heat.

When the water boils turn off the heat. Add the zucchini to the hot water. Stir and let stand for 1 minute.

Drain and add to a mixing bowl with the shallot, tomato, lime juice, olive oil, maple syrup, salt, pepper,
red pepper flakes, chili powder and cilantro.

Stir well and chill.

*"Sharing food with another human being is an
intimate act that should not be indulged in lightly."*
M. F. K. Fisher

The refrigerator light goes on...
This is a fantastic side dish for your tacos or as
a topping for your taco salad. Use wherever you
might use a salsa!

Nutrition Facts

Serving size	about 1 cup
Servings	4
Calories 70	Calories from Fat 34
	(% Daily Value)
Total Fat 3 g	(5 %)
Saturated Fat 0 g	(2 %)
Trans Fat 0 g	
Monounsaturated Fat 2 g	
Cholesterol 0 mg	(0 %)
Sodium 162 mg	(6 %)
Total Carbohydrates 9 g	(2 %)
Dietary Fiber 2 g	(6 %)
Sugars 4 g	
Protein 1 g	
Vitamin A 19 %	Vitamin C 52 %
Calcium 1 %	Iron 6 %
Vitamin K 13 mcg	
Potassium 461 mg	Magnesium 28 mg

Zucchini Salad

Servings = 4
Serving size = about 1 1/2 cups

This recipe can easily be multiplied. This recipe keeps well for about 48 hours.

2 Tbsp.	olive oil
2 Tbsp.	balsamic vinegar
2 Tbsp.	maple syrup
1/4 tsp.	salt
to taste	fresh ground black pepper
1 tsp.	dried marjoram
1 lb.	zucchini (cut into medium dice)
8 ounces	grape tomatoes
4 Tbsp.	pine nuts

Whisk together the olive oil, balsamic vinegar, maple syrup, salt, pepper and marjoram. Place in the refrigerator while cutting the zucchini.

Cut the zucchini into medium dice. This should be about 1/4 inch cubes.

Toss the zucchini, tomatoes and pine nuts together in the vinaigrette. Chill well before serving.

"To remember a successful salad is generally to remember a successful dinner; at all events, the perfect dinner necessarily includes the perfect salad."

George Ellwanger, Gastronomist

The refrigerator light goes on...
I love this little salad. It's quick and easy and really tasty. You can use yellow squash as well or combine the two for great color. It makes a great side dish for almost any soup and you have the perfect dinner.

Nutrition Facts

Serving size	about 1 1/2 cups
Servings	4

Calories 178	Calories from Fat 111
	(% Daily Value)
Total Fat 13 g	(20 %)
Saturated Fat 1 g	(7 %)
Trans Fat 0 g	
Monounsaturated Fat 7 g	
Cholesterol 41 mg	(14 %)
Sodium 162 mg	(7 %)
Total Carbohydrates 15 g	(5 %)
Dietary Fiber 2 g	(9 %)
Sugars 11 g	
Protein 3 g	
Vitamin A 14 %	Vitamin C 44 %
Calcium 4 %	Iron 7 %
Vitamin K 19 mcg	
Potassium 508 mg	Magnesium 49 mg

Zucchini with Sun Dried Tomatoes

Servings = 2
Serving size = about 1 1/2 cups

This recipe can easily be multiplied but does not make very good leftovers.

1 tsp.	olive oil
2 medium	sun dried tomato slices
1 Tbsp.	pinenuts
2 medium	zucchini (large dice)
1/4 tsp.	salt
1/4 tsp.	dried thyme leaves
to taste	fresh ground black pepper

Place a large skillet over medium heat. Add the olive oil, and after about a minute, add the sun dried tomato and pinenuts.

Cook, stirring frequently, for about 5 minutes. Reduce the heat if necessary so that the pinenuts don't brown too much - they should be a light golden brown.

Add the zucchini, salt, thyme and pepper. Increase the heat to medium high. Cook, tossing frequently, until the zucchini just begins to brown on all sides and is slightly soft.

"I used to visit and revisit it a dozen times a day, and stand in deep contemplation over my vegetable progeny with a love that nobody could share or conceive of who had never taken part in the process of creation. It was one of the most bewitching sights in the world to observe a hill of beans thrusting aside the soil, or a rose of early peas just peeping forth sufficiently to trace a line of delicate green."

Nathaniel Hawthorne, Author

The refrigerator light goes on...
This goes well with almost any dish, but it's especially good with a steak or roasted pork main course. The zucchini is simple to prep. Cut the stem end off and make three slices lengthways so you have 4 slices. Stack two slices and cut lengthways three times again. Do this with all four slices and then cut crossways for a large dice.

Nutrition Facts

Serving size	about 1 1/2 cups
Servings	2
Calories 84	Calories from Fat 47
	(% Daily Value)
Total Fat 5 g	(8 %)
Saturated Fat 1 g	(3 %)
Trans Fat 0 g	
Monounsaturated Fat 2 g	
Cholesterol 0 mg	(0 %)
Sodium 352 mg	(15 %)
Total Carbohydrates 8 g	(3 %)
Dietary Fiber 3 g	(10 %)
Sugars 4 g	
Protein 3 g	
Vitamin A 8 %	Vitamin C 57 %
Calcium 3 %	Iron 7 %
Vitamin K 15 mcg	
Potassium 607 mg	Magnesium 47 mg

Butternut Squash Risotto

4 **45 min.**

Serving size = about 2 cups
This recipe can easily be multiplied. Leftovers are good. Reheat gently.

1 – 2 lb.	butternut squash
	spray olive oil
2 tsp.	extra virgin olive oil
1 large	leek
1/2 medium	red onion (diced)
1 cup	arborio rice
3 cups	water
1 cup	low sodium chicken broth
1/4 cup	dry sherry
1/4 tsp.	salt
	fresh ground black pepper to taste
1/4 tsp.	ground paprika
1 1/2 ounces	Parmigiano-Reggiano (grated)
1 Tbsp	Italian parsley leaves

Preheat the oven to 325°F.

Slice the squash lengthwise and remove the seeds. Spray lightly with olive oil and place in the preheated oven, cut side up. Roast the squash for about 1 hour, until slightly tender.

Remove from the oven and let cool. The squash will have a small amount of liquid in the cavity. After it is cool, drain the liquid and place the squash on a cutting board, cut side down.

Gently peel the skin away from the squash. Slice across the squash parallel to the cutting board, dividing into three slices. Keep the shape of the squash intact. Slice lengthwise at about 1/4 inch intervals and then crosswise, so as to divide into 1/2 inch cubes. Set aside.

Slice the root off of the leek. Slice the leek in half, separating the white from the green tops. Clean the green tops under running water and slice very thin. Slice the white part of the leek very thin lengthwise and clean well.

Heat the olive oil in a large sauce pan over high heat and add the green part of the leek. Reduce the heat to medium-high and cook very slowly. Stir frequently.

When the leek is wilted, add the white part of the leek and the diced red onion. Reduce the heat to medium and cook for about five minutes, until the onions begin to soften.

Place the rice in the pan with the onions and leeks and stir for about 3 minutes. Add two cups of water, the chicken stock, sherry, salt and pepper. Cook over medium-high heat stirring frequently. Add the remaining water, 1 cup at a time.

Add the ground paprika and continue cooking. The rice will take about 20 to 25 minutes to cook and may require more water be added. Stir frequently, using about 1/2 cup of water at a time as needed, until the rice is soft but not mushy and there is a small amount of creamy sauce.

Stir in the Parmigiano-Reggiano until it is melted and then gently fold in the diced butternut squash and parsley.

The refrigerator light goes on...
Risotto is one of my favorite ingredients because it makes an amazingly rich sauce as it cooks, without having to use too much fat. It is the ultimate healthy ingredient. It's easy and quick and should always be in your pantry.

Nutrition Facts

Serving size	About 2 cups risotto
Servings	4
Calories 394	Calories from Fat 52
	(% Daily Value)
Total Fat 6 g	(9 %)
Saturated Fat 2 g	(11 %)
Trans Fat 0 g	
Monounsaturated Fat 3 g	
Cholesterol 7 mg	(2 %)
Sodium 348 mg	(14 %)
Total Carbohydrates 73 g	(24 %)
Dietary Fiber 7 g	(26 %)
Sugars 8 g	
Protein 11 g	
Vitamin A 487 %	Vitamin C 87 %
Calcium 25 %	Iron 25 %
Vitamin K 30 mcg	
Potassium 970 mg	Magnesium 103 mg
Potassium 387 mg	Magnesium 15 mg

Chalupas

Servings = 2
Serving size = 3 chalupas

This recipe is easily multiplied several times or cut in half. This recipe also requires making Guacamole (recipe included). Once assembled, the chalupas do not keep well, mostly because the tortillas fall apart.

6	soft corn tortillas
1/2 cup	canned refried beans
2 ounces	reduced fat Monterey Jack cheese (shredded)
6	leaves Romaine lettuce (shredded fine)
1 large	tomato (coarsely chopped)
1/2 cup	cilantro leaves (chopped)
6 Tbsp	Guacamole
	fresh ground black pepper (to taste)

Preheat the oven to 325°F.

Spread the refried beans equally across the six tortillas. Sprinkle with the cheese and place in the oven.

When the cheese is just melted, remove the tortillas from the oven and top with the lettuce, tomato, cilantro, pepper, guacamole and salsa.

Serve.

"Do good and don't worry to whom.
Mexican Proverb

The refrigerator light goes on...
I love chalupas, and like tacos and enchiladas, there are endless varieties. This recipe is based on a Mexican restaurant that I used to eat at in Houston 20 years ago. Since then I have loved the refried beans topped with cheese, all warm and soft topped with fresh salad. You can strike any variation that you like. I particularly like a base of salsa verde instead of the refried black beans.

The Nutrition Facts are based on you using canned refried black beans which have waaay too much sodium, but I wanted you to see the worst case. A half cup of Old El Paso Traditional Refried Beans has a whopping 580 mg in a half cup of refried beans. There are alternatives. The Dr. Gourmet recipe for Refried Black Beans (recipe included) will save you about 200 mg sodium per serving.

Amy's offers good alternatives that come in at only 200 mg in a 1/2 cup serving, and their refried black beans are really great with this recipe.

Nutrition Facts

Serving size	3 chalupas
Servings	2
Calories 324	Calories from Fat 136
	(% Daily Value)
Total Fat 16g	(24%)
Saturated Fat 5g	(27%)
Trans Fat 0 g	
Monounsaturated Fat 18g	
Cholesterol 18mg	(6%)
Sodium 584mg	(24%)
Total Carbohydrates 34g	(11%)
Dietary Fiber 10g	(41%)
Sugars 4g	
Protein 15g	
Vitamin A 30%	Vitamin C 36%
Calcium 27%	Iron 13%
Vitamin K 35 mcg	
Potassium 846 mg	Magnesium 86 mg

Chile Rellenos

2 **60 min.**

Serving size = 2 peppers

This recipe can be multiplied. The cooked chile rellenos do not keep well.

1 small	dried chipotle chili
1 tsp	grapeseed oil
1 medium	white onion (minced)
1/4 tsp	ground cumin
4 medium	poblano peppers
3 ounces	reduced-fat Monterey jack cheese (shredded)
4 Tbsp	fresh cilantro
1 large	egg
1 large	egg white
1 Tbsp	Dijon mustard
4 ounces	plain melba toast
1/4 tsp	ground cumin
1/4 tsp	salt
1/4 tsp	ground black pepper
1/8 tsp	cayenne pepper

Place a steamer basket in a small sauce pan with about a cup of water in the bottom of it. Heat the steamer over high heat and place the chipotle inside. When it is soft, move it to a cutting board and carefully remove the seeds. Avoid touching the pepper with your hands. If you do, wash your hands well.

Mince the chipotle and set aside.

Place the canola oil in a large non-stick skillet and heat over medium heat. Add the onion and cook slowly until translucent. Add the minced chipotle and cook for another two minutes. Remove from the heat and chill in the refrigerator for about an hour.

Preheat oven to broil. Place the poblano peppers in the oven and roast them, turning by 1/4 turn about every three minutes. The skin of the chili should begin to turn black. After the skin is blackened, remove the peppers from the oven and place in a brown paper bag.

After about 30 minutes, the peppers should be cool. Remove them from the paper bag and gently peel the thin skin from the pepper. Using the point of a knife, make a slit down the long side of each pepper. Gently remove the core and seeds from the inside, trying to keep the pepper whole.

After the cooked onion is cool, toss it together with the cilantro and shredded cheese. Form the cheese into 8 small cylinders. Place the cylinders inside the peppers and reform the poblanos to resemble whole peppers.

Place the egg, egg white and mustard in a small bowl. Whisk until smooth.

In a food processor, place the melba toast, ground cumin, salt, black pepper and cayenne pepper and process until small bread crumbs. Leave some pieces about the size of currants.

Preheat oven to 400°F.

Coat the peppers with the egg and mustard mixture and then coat with the melba toast crumbs. After all of them are coated, place on a non-stick cookie sheet then put them into the oven. Bake for about 15 minutes. Spray lightly with spray oil and turn at about 7 minutes.

Nutrition Facts

Serving size	2 peppers
Servings	2
Calories 484	Calories from Fat 146
	(% Daily Value)
Total Fat 16g	(25%)
Saturated Fat 7g	(36%)
Trans Fat 0 g	
Monounsaturated Fat 4g	
Cholesterol 133mg	(34%)
Sodium 695mg	(29%)
Total Carbohydrates 59g	(20%)
Dietary Fiber 8g	(32%)
Sugars 8g	
Protein 26g	
Vitamin A 23%	Vitamin C 214%
Calcium 41%	Iron 23%
Vitamin K 19 mcg	
Potassium 626 mg	Magnesium 79 mg

Chilled White Bean Soup with Sun Dried Tomatoes

4　**90 min.**

Serving size = about 1 1/2 cups

This recipe can be multplied and makes great left-overs.

2 ounces	sun dried tomatoes
5 cups	water
2 Tbsp	green bell pepper (finely diced)
1 Tbsp	shallot (minced)
2 tsp	olive oil
1 medium	white onion (diced)
2 medium	ribs celery (diced)
2 15 ounce cans	no salt added white beans (drained and rinsed)
1/4 tsp	salt
to taste	fresh ground black pepper
3 Tbsp	fresh oregano

Place the sun dried tomatoes in a small sauce pan with 1 cup water. Place the sauce pan over high heat and when it begins to boil reduce the heat to low and simmer until all the water has evaporated.

When the tomatoes are cooked allow them to cool slightly and then mince.

Toss together with the peppers, shallot and 1 teaspoon of the olive oil. Chill.

While the tomatoes are cooking place the other 1 teaspoon olive oil in a large sauce pan over medium high heat. Add the diced onion and cook for about 4 minutes.

Add the celery and cook, stirring frequently, for about 4 minutes.

Add the beans, salt and pepper with the remaining 4 cups water. Stir, let come to a slow boil and then reduce the heat to low. Cover and simmer for 45 minutes.

Let the soup cool for about 20 minutes, add the oregano and puree with a immersion blender or in a blender.

Chill.

Serve the soup chilled topped with the sun dried tomato compote.

"Think of New York as a puree and the rest of the United States as vegetable soup."
Spalding Gray, Author

The refrigerator light goes on...
This is so light and refreshing for summer but at the same time filling and satisfying. Serve with a side salad and a whole grain or gluten-free roll for the perfect meal on a hot day.

Nutrition Facts

Serving size	about 1 1/2 cups
Servings	4
Calories 272	Calories from Fat 33
	(% Daily Value)
Total Fat 3g	(9%)
Saturated Fat <1g	(2%)
Trans Fat 0 g	
Monounsaturated Fat 2g	
Cholesterol 0mg	(0%)
Sodium 460mg	(20%)
Total Carbohydrates 49g	(16%)
Dietary Fiber 17g	(60%)
Sugars 5g	
Protein 22g	
Vitamin A 8%	Vitamin C 24%
Calcium 16%	Iron 27%
Vitamin K 19 mcg	
Potassium 1155 mg	Magnesium 109 mg

Cream of Potato Soup with Roasted Garlic

4 **30 min.**

Serving Size = about 2 cups

This recipe can be multiplied. This recipe requires making Roasted Garlic (recipe included). Makes great leftovers.

1 tsp	olive oil
1 small	white onion (diced)
12 ounces	Idaho potato (peeled and cubed)
4 cups	water
1 cup	2% milk
1	bulb roasted garlic
1/2 tsp	salt
to taste	fresh ground black pepper
12 ounces	Yukon Gold potato (peeled and cubed)
4 ounces	smoked gouda (shredded)

Place the olive oil in a medium sauce pan over medium heat. Add the onion and cook for about 4 minutes, stirring frequently. Do not allow the onion to brown.

Add the Idaho potato and water. Reduce the heat to medium and simmer for about 30 minutes until the potatoes are soft.

Add the milk, roasted garlic, salt and pepper. Using a blender or stick blender puree until smooth.

Return the soup to medium heat and add the Yukon gold potatoes. Cook for about 20 minutes until the potatoes are soft.

Serve each bowl of soup topped with one ounce of smoked gouda.

"You can never have enough garlic. With enough garlic, you can eat 'The New York Times.'"
Morley Safer, Journalist

The refrigerator light goes on...
On a cold Fall or Winter night there's nothing more comforting than a bowl of potato soup. This recipe is so savory with the garlic and smoked gouda and makes the perfect meal with a simple side salad.

Nutrition Facts

Serving size	about 1 1/2 cups
Servings	4
Calories 272	Calories from Fat 33
	(% Daily Value)
Total Fat 3g	(9%)
Saturated Fat <1g	(2%)
Trans Fat 0 g	
Monounsaturated Fat 2g	
Cholesterol 0mg	(0%)
Sodium 460mg	(20%)
Total Carbohydrates 49g	(16%)
Dietary Fiber 17g	(60%)
Sugars 5g	
Protein 22g	
Vitamin A 8%	Vitamin C 24%
Calcium 16%	Iron 27%
Vitamin K 19 mcg	
Potassium 1155 mg	Magnesium 109 mg

Curried Cauliflower

3 **30 min.**

Serving size = about 2 cups (8 ounces cauliflower)

This recipe can easily be multiplied. Leftovers are great. Reheat gently. Serve over jasmine or brown rice.

1 tsp	olive oil
1 tsp	curry powder
1/2 tsp	ground cumin
1/2	10 ounce package frozen diced onions
1	16 ounce package frozen cauliflower
1 15 ounce can	no salt added diced tomatoes
1/4 tsp	salt
to taste	fresh ground black pepper
1 15 ounce can	no salt added chick peas (garbanzos)
1/4 cup	2% milk
1/2 cup	frozen peas

Place the olive oil in a large skillet over medium heat. Add the cumin and curry powder and as the pan heats up. Stir frequently.

When the pan is hot add the onions and the cauliflower. Cook for about 7 minutes and add the tomatoes, salt and pepper. Stir well and cook for about 5 minutes. Add the chick peas and milk and cook for about 7 minutes.

Add the peas and cook for about 3 - 5 minutes. Serve over Brown Rice.

"Without the curry, boiled rice can be very dull."
C. Northcote Parkinson, Author

The refrigerator light goes on...
I was surprised when I made this recipe. I had thought that it would make 2 servings but along with the brown rice it is so filling that it really is three servings. Even then it is amazingly filling.

The key to enhancing the flavor is to sauté the curry powder in the olive oil for a bit to soften the flavor. Add the cauliflower and then the other ingredients.

Nutrition Facts

Serving size	about 2 cups
Servings	3

Calories 258	Calories from Fat 40
	(% Daily Value)
Total Fat 4g	(7%)
Saturated Fat 1g	(2%)
Trans Fat 0 g	
Monounsaturated Fat 2g	
Cholesterol 2mg	(1%)
Sodium 298mg	(12%)
Total Carbohydrates 45g	(15%)
Dietary Fiber 13g	(53%)
Sugars 15g	
Protein 14g	
Vitamin A 14%	Vitamin C 149%
Calcium 16%	Iron 28%
Vitamin K 38 mcg	
Potassium 1074 mg	Magnesium 92 mg

Curried Eggplant

3 **30 min.**

Serving size = 6 ounces eggplant with sauce and cheese

This recipe is easily multiplied. Reheat gently. Serve with Jasmine Rice, Coconut Rice, or Brown Rice.

2 tsp	olive oil
2 tsp	curry powder
1 tsp	ground coriander
1/2 tsp	ground cumin
1/8 tsp	red pepper flakes (optional)
1 small	onion (diced)
1 clove	garlic (sliced)
1 15 ounce can	diced tomatoes
1/4 tsp	salt
to taste	fresh ground black pepper
	spray olive oil
1 1/2 lb	eggplant (sliced into rounds about 1/4 inch thick)
1/4 cup	dried pumpkin seeds
4 ounces	paneer cheese (cut into small cubes)

Place the olive oil in a large skillet over medium heat. Add the curry powder, coriander, cumin and cayenne and cook, stirring frequently. Let the oil bubble but don't let the pan get too hot – reduce the heat if the oil is bubbling too much. Cook for about 3 minutes.

Add the onion and garlic and cook, stirring frequently, for about 5 minutes until the onions begin to soften. Add the tomatoes, salt and pepper. Cook for about 10 minutes and remove from the heat. Let cool and then puree until smooth. Set aside.

Clean the skillet and place over medium high heat. Spray with olive oil and add the eggplant slices. Cook on each side until slightly browned. Lightly spray with olive oil as needed. As the slices are cooked, remove them to paper towels.

Preheat the oven to 325°F. Line a 9 inch oblong pyrex dish with foil.

When all the eggplant slices are cooked, place a layer of eggplant slices in the bottom of the pyrex dish. Top with 1/2 of the curry sauce and then 1/2 of the pumpkin seeds. Place a second layer of eggplant on

top of the sauce. Use the remaining curry sauce and pumpkin seeds to cover the eggplant.

Place the dish in the oven and cook uncovered for 10 minutes.

Remove and sprinkle the cheese over the eggplant, then return the dish to the oven. Leave the dish in the oven for about 5 minutes, until the cheese is melted.

"I realize that when I met you at the turkey curry buffet, I was unforgivably rude, and wearing a reindeer jumper."
Helen Fielding, Author of *Bridget Jones Diary*

The refrigerator light goes on...
Paneer is a great cheese, especially for those on a low sodium diet. It is an Indian cheese that is sort of a cross between mozzarella and tofu. It has a good firm texture and soft milk flavor. The best part is that most are made with very little salt. It used to be hard to find but is now widely available in many groceries. If you can't find it, use fresh mozzarella, but add only 1/8 tsp. salt.

Nutrition Facts

Serving size	about 1 1/2 cups
Servings	4

Calories 272	Calories from Fat 33
	(% Daily Value)
Total Fat 3g	(9%)
Saturated Fat <1g	(2%)
Trans Fat 0 g	
Monounsaturated Fat 2g	
Cholesterol 0mg	(0%)
Sodium 460mg	(20%)
Total Carbohydrates 49g	(16%)
Dietary Fiber 17g	(60%)
Sugars 5g	
Protein 22g	

Vitamin A 8%	Vitamin C 24%
Calcium 16%	Iron 27%
Vitamin K 19 mcg	
Potassium 1155 mg	Magnesium 109 mg

Eggplant Curry with Rice Noodles

2 **30 min.**

Serving size = 1 1/2 ounces noodles with veggies

This recipe can easily be multiplied. This recipe does not make very good leftovers.

1 tsp	olive oil
1 small	onion (sliced)
4 ounces	crimini mushrooms (quartered)
1 large	carrot (peeled and cubed)
1	eggplant (about 1/2 pound) (cut into large cubes)
1 tsp	curry powder
1/4 cup	light coconut milk
1/8 tsp	salt
1/2 tsp	sugar
1 3/4 cup	water
to taste	fresh ground black pepper
1/3 cup	raisins
3 ounces	paneer cheese (cubed)
3 ounces	rice noodles

Mix together the water, curry powder, coconut milk, sugar, salt and pepper in a small bowl. Set aside.

Place the olive oil in a large non-stick skillet (one with a lid) over medium-high heat. Add the onion and cook, tossing frequently, for two minutes.

Add the carrot, eggplant and mushrooms, toss together, and cover. Reduce heat to medium. Cook for 6-8 minutes, tossing occasionally, until the eggplant begins to soften.

Add the curry mixture, rice noodles and raisin, cover, and allow to cook for 5 minutes. Stir and add paneer. Toss and recover.

Cook for another 3 – 5 minutes until the noodles are done.

"I doubt that the imagination can be suppressed. If you truly eradicated it in a child, he would grow up to be an eggplant."
Ursula K. LeGuin, Author

The refrigerator light goes on...
I love cooking with paneer. It's a medium fat cheese with 8 grams of fat in a serving, but there's no sodium added. While this makes for a mild cheese, I think that it works as a perfect complement to full flavored sauces and spicy foods.

Nutrition Facts

Serving size	1 1/2 ounces noodles with veggies
Servings	2
Calories 542	Calories from Fat 140
	(% Daily Value)
Total Fat 16g	(25%)
Saturated Fat 9g	(45%)
Trans Fat 0 g	
Monounsaturated Fat 5g	
Cholesterol 29mg	(10%)
Sodium 479mg	(20%)
Total Carbohydrates 87g	(29%)
Dietary Fiber 8g	(34%)
Sugars 33g	
Protein 17g	
Vitamin A 128%	Vitamin C 15%
Calcium 39%	Iron 14%
Vitamin K 14 mcg	
Potassium 1097 mg	Magnesium 446 mg

Eggplant Lasagna

4 **90 min.**

Serving size = 1/4 lasagna

This recipe can be multiplied up to 4 times, but you'll need several pans. This recipe makes great leftovers, and like many lasagnas, is even better the next day.

2 tsp	olive oil
2 cloves	garlic (minced)
1 large	onion (diced)
1 lb	crimini mushrooms (sliced)
2 15 ounce can	no salt added diced tomatoes
1/4 tsp	salt
to taste	fresh ground black pepper
2 tsp	dried basil
1 tsp	dried oregano
1/2 tsp	dried thyme
	spray oil
1 1/2 lbs	eggplant (thinly sliced into rounds)
8 ounces	low-moisture part-skim mozzarella slices

Place the olive oil in a large skillet over medium high heat.

Add the garlic and cook for about 2 minutes. Stir frequently.

Add the onion and cook for about 4 minutes. Stir frequently.

Add the mushrooms and cook for about 10 minutes until well browned.

Add the tomatoes, salt, pepper, basil, oregano and thyme. Stir and reduce the heat to medium.

Cover and simmer for 10 minutes. Stir occasionally.

Uncover and simmer for another 15 minutes. Stir occasionally.

Preheat the oven to 325°F.

Line a 9"x12" rectangular Pyrex dish with aluminum foil. Spray lightly with oil.

Place a layer of 1/2 of the eggplant slices in the bottom of the pan. Top with 1/2 of the sauce.
Place another layer of the remaining eggplant in the pan and then top with the remaining sauce.

Cover the lasagna with foil. Place the pan in the oven and cook for 30 minutes. Increase the heat to 375°F and cook for another 30 minutes.

Remove the foil and top with the sliced mozzarella.

Cook for another 10 minutes. Serve.

"I prepare the vegetables with a wide range of herbs, spices and such."
Graham Kerr, The Galloping Gourmet

The refrigerator light goes on...
This recipe was designed to use layers of eggplant in place of the traditional strips of lasagna pasta. One thing to keep in mind with this recipe is to cook the sauce long enough so that it is fairly thick. The eggplant will give up a fair amount of water while baking, and if the sauce is too thin, the "lasagna" won't hold together well.

Nutrition Facts

Serving size	1/4 lasagna
Servings	4

Calories 308	Calories from Fat 128
	(% Daily Value)
Total Fat 13g	(22%)
Saturated Fat 7g	(29%)
Trans Fat 0 g	
Monounsaturated Fat 5g	
Cholesterol 31mg	(10%)
Sodium 466mg	(19%)
Total Carbohydrates 8g	(2%)
Dietary Fiber 9g	(31%)
Sugars 10g	
Protein 22g	
Vitamin A 9%	Vitamin C 30%
Calcium 54%	Iron 13%
Vitamin K 21 mcg	
Potassium 1235 mg	Magnesium 67 mg

Eggplant Parmesan

2 **60 min.**

Serving size = a lot

This recipe can easily be multiplied. This keeps well for about 48 hours in the fridge.

1 cup	water
2	8 ounce eggplants (sliced lengthwise in 1/2 inch slices)
2 ounces	plain no salt added melba toast
1/4 tsp	dried basil
1/4 tsp	dried oregano
1/4 tsp	garlic powder
1/8 tsp	fresh ground black pepper
2	egg whites
4 ounces	fresh mozzarella
8 large	leaves fresh basil
1 cup	marinara sauce
1 ounce	Parmigiano-Reggiano (grated)

Place the water in a large stock pot fitted with a steamer. Heat over high heat. When the water is boiling place the eggplant slices in the steamer for 10 minutes.

Remove to a cutting board to cool.

While the eggplant is steaming place the melba toast, basil, oregano, garlic powder and pepper in a food processor and process until fine crumbs.

Preheat the oven to 350°F.

Whisk the egg whites until frothy.

When the eggplant is cool coat each slice one at a time with egg white. Let excess eggwhite drip off and then dredge in the bread crumb mixture. As each slice is coated place on a non-stick cookie sheet.

Place the coated eggplant in the oven and bake for 10 minutes on each side.

Remove and layer the eggplant with slices of mozzarella and fresh basil in an au gratin or similar dish -- slice of eggplant, slice of mozzarella, basil, slice of eggplant, slice of mozzarella, etc.. It's OK if the layers are on their side or not just perfect. Each au gratin dish should hold one serving.

Top the eggplant layers with 1/2 cup of marinara sauce and place in oven for 5 minutes. Top with the Parmigiano-reggiano and bake for another 5 minutes.

"And my baby cooks her Eggplant,
Bout 19 different ways.
Sometimes I just have it raw with Mayonnaise."
Michael Franks, Singer/Songwriter

The refrigerator light goes on...
This is a time consuming recipe but oh, so worth it!

It is something that you are going to have for a special occasion as it will take about an hour (or a little more) on a Saturday afternoon to make. It is very rewarding. It is higher in fat and sodium than many Dr. Gourmet recipes, but it can still be part of your diet occasionally and should because Eggplant Parmesan is so great. You can feel better because this is chock full of great things like fiber, Vitamin A, iron, calcium and Vitamin C.

Nutrition Facts

Serving size	a lot
Servings	2

Calories 451	Calories from Fat 155
	(% Daily Value)
Total Fat 18g	(27%)
Saturated Fat 10g	(49%)
Trans Fat 0 g	
Monounsaturated Fat 5g	
Cholesterol 43mg	(14%)
Sodium 1069mg	(45%)
Total Carbohydrates 45g	(15%)
Dietary Fiber 11g	(43%)
Sugars 11g	
Protein 30g	
Vitamin A 14%	Vitamin C 24%
Calcium 66%	Iron 19%
Vitamin K 22 mcg	
Potassium 943 mg	Magnesium 87 mg

Eggplant Risotto

2 **30 min.**

Serving size = about 2 cups

This recipe can easily be multiplied and makes great leftovers.

2 tsp	olive oil
1 clove	garlic (sliced)
1 small	onion (sliced)
1 large	eggplant (cut into 1 inch cubes)
1/4 tsp	dried tarragon
1/2 tsp	dried oregano
1/2 tsp	dried basil
1/2 tsp	dried rosemary
1/2 cup	arborio rice
to taste	fresh ground black pepper
2 cups	low sodium chicken or vegetable broth
3 cups	water
4 ounces	cherry or grape tomatoes
1 ounce	Parmigiano-Reggiano (grated)
2 ounces	fresh mozzarella (cut into small dice)

Place the olive oil in a medium sized skillet over medium-high heat. Add the garlic and onion and cook for about one minute. Stir frequently.

Add the eggplant and cook, stirring frequently. Adjust the heat as needed to keep the eggplant from burning but turn a nut brown.

Add the dried tarragon, oregano, basil, rosemary and arborio rice and cook for about one minute.

Add the pepper, chicken stock, water and tomatoes. Stir once and reduce the heat until the rice is simmering. Cook for about 15 minutes until the rice is tender.

Add the parmesan and stir until blended. Serve the risotto topped with the fresh mozzarella cubes.

"Washington, DC is to lying what Wisconsin is to cheese."

Dennis Miller, Comedian

The refrigerator light goes on...
I was having a discussion recently about how to create great low-sodium recipes and this is a great example. There's no added salt but there are a lot of salty flavors. The parmesan and mozzarella add a lot of this. The other key is that there are so many umami flavors – onions, eggplant and the cheeses. The blend of these flavors are enhanced by the herbs. The result is that there's less need for added salt. Best of all, the rich creaminess of the risotto makes for a lovely sauce.

Nutrition Facts

Serving size	1/4 lasagna
Servings	4

Calories 308	Calories from Fat 128
	(% Daily Value)
Total Fat 13g	(22%)
Saturated Fat 7g	(29%)
Trans Fat 0 g	
Monounsaturated Fat 5g	
Cholesterol 31mg	(10%)
Sodium 466mg	(19%)
Total Carbohydrates 8g	(2%)
Dietary Fiber 9g	(31%)
Sugars 10g	
Protein 22g	
Vitamin A 9%	Vitamin C 30%
Calcium 54%	Iron 13%
Vitamin K 21 mcg	
Potassium 1235 mg	Magnesium 67 mg

Fettuccine Alfredo

2 **30 min.**

Serving size = 2 ounces pasta with sauce

This recipe can be multiplied up to 5 times and re-quires making Roasted Garlic (recipe included). Left-overs are fair at best. Serve with Herbed Zucchini or Parmesan Squash (recipes included.)

1 tsp	extra virgin olive oil
2 cloves	roasted garlic (minced)
2 tsp	all purpose white flour
3/4 cup	2% milk (chilled)
1 ounce	semi-soft goat cheese
1 ounce	Parmigiano-Reggiano (grated)
4 quarts	water
4 ounces	whole wheat fettuccine
1 Tbsp	parsley (minced)

Heat the olive oil in a ten-inch non-stick skillet over medium heat and add the roasted garlic. Cook very slowly and stir frequently. Do not allow the garlic to brown or it will become bitter.

Add the flour slowly and cook for about one minute. Stir continuously to blend the oil and flour. The mix-ture will be like coarse corn meal. Cook gently so the mixture doesn't brown.

Slowly add the cold milk whisking to keep the sauce from forming clumps. Blend in all of the milk until the sauce is smooth and begins to thicken.

Add the goat cheese and whisk as it melts. When the sauce is smooth add the Parmigiano-Reggiano and whisk as it melts until the sauce is creamy. Reduce the heat to very low.

In a large pot heat the water to a boil. Add the fettuc-cine and cook until just tender (about 12 – 15 minutes for dried pasta). Drain well and then add the pasta to the sauce, tossing to coat thoroughly. Sprinkle the minced parsley over the top and serve.

"Tomatoes and oregano make it Italian; wine and tarragon make it French. Sour cream makes it Russian; lemon and cinnamon make it Greek. Soy sauce makes it Chinese; garlic makes it good."
Alice May Brock, Owner of
Alice's Restaurant

The refrigerator light goes on...
Keep in mind a serving of any pasta is two ounces. I prefer to use the best quality Parmesan cheese and grate it fresh. By using the best quality ingredients you don't need as much to get maximum flavor.

Nutrition Facts

Serving size	2 ounces pasta with sauce
Servings	2
Calories 389	Calories from Fat 107
	(% Daily Value)
Total Fat 12g	(19%)
Saturated Fat 6g	(30%)
Trans Fat 0 g	
Monounsaturated Fat 5g	
Cholesterol 23mg	(8%)
Sodium 337mg	(14%)
Total Carbohydrates 53g	(18%)
Dietary Fiber 5g	(20%)
Sugars 5g	
Protein 20g	
Vitamin A 7%	Vitamin C 11%
Calcium 36%	Iron 16%
Vitamin K 33 mcg	
Potassium 354 mg	Magnesium 107 mg

Fettuccine with Olive Oil and Garlic

2 **30 min.**

Serving size = 2 ounces pasta with sauce

This recipe can easily be multiplied but does not make very good leftovers.

2 quarts	water
4 ounces	whole wheat fettuccine
1 Tbsp	extra virgin olive oil
3 cloves	garlic (minced)
6 large	pitted black olives – like kalamata (coarsely chopped)
1/4 cup	white wine
1/8 tsp	salt
to taste	fresh ground black pepper
2 medium	tomatoes (seeded and cut into strips)
1 Tbsp	extra virgin olive oil
8 large	leaves fresh basil (chiffonade)
1 ounce	Parmigiano-Reggiano (grated)

"There are five elements: earth, air, fire, water and garlic."

Louis Diat, Chef

The refrigerator light goes on...
Cooking the garlic and olives together slowly will infuse the flavors of both into the olive oil. The key is to not let the garlic brown or it will turn bitter. You can try other ingredients. Use shallots or leeks instead of the garlic, for example. Green beans or peas are fantastic in place of the tomatoes. Try this recipe changing one ingredient at a time to make your own favorite.

Place the water in a large stock pot over high heat.

While the water is heating place the first tablespoon olive oil in a large skillet over medium-low heat. Add the minced garlic and chopped olives. Adjust the heat to low and cook the garlic and olives slowly so that the garlic doesn't brown.

When the water is boiling add the fettuccine. Cook, stirring occasionally.

While the pasta is cooking continue to cook the garlic and olives. When the pasta is done add transfer it to the pan with the olive oil. Grab the fettuccine using tongs and let it drain slightly before placing it in the skillet. Don't be too concerned that some of the pasta water may transfer.

When all the fettuccine is in the skillet increase the heat to medium-high and add the white wine, salt and pepper. Toss the mixture and as the liquid in the pan begins to evaporate add the tomatoes and the second tablespoon of olive oil.

Cook for another 1 - 2 minutes and add the basil. Toss and serve topped with the grated cheese.

Nutrition Facts

Serving size	2 ounces pasta with sauce
Servings	2
Calories 472	Calories from Fat 175
	(% Daily Value)
Total Fat 20g	(31%)
Saturated Fat 5g	(23%)
Trans Fat 0 g	
Monounsaturated Fat 12g	
Cholesterol 10mg	(3%)
Sodium 465mg	(19%)
Total Carbohydrates 53g	(18%)
Dietary Fiber 7g	(28%)
Sugars 4g	
Protein 15g	
Vitamin A 26%	Vitamin C 30%
Calcium 24%	Iron 21%
Vitamin K 30 mcg	
Potassium 501 mg	Magnesium 111 mg

Lentils and Eggs

2 **60 min.**

Serving size = about 2 cups lentils with 1 egg

This recipe can easily be multiplied but does not make good leftovers.

1/2 cup	green lentils
4 cups	water
1 Tbsp	olive oil
4 ounces	crimini mushrooms (sliced)
1 large	onion (diced)
1/4 tsp	salt
to taste	fresh ground black pepper
1/2 tsp	paprika
2 tsp	dried sage
2 large	eggs

Place the lentils in a bowl with 2 cups of the water. Stir and let stand for 30 minutes.

Place 1 teaspoon of the olive oil in a skillet over medium high heat. Add the mushrooms and cook, tossing frequently, sweating the mushrooms until they are well browned and caramelized.

Remove the mushrooms to a plate.

Place the other 2 teaspoons olive oil in the skillet and add the diced onion. Cook, stirring frequently, until softened. Add the lentils with the two cups water they have been soaking in.

Add the salt, pepper, paprika and sage.

Simmer over medium high heat. Add water 1/2 cup at a time cooking for about 20 – 25 minutes. Stir occasionally. As the lentils get soft add less water.

When the lentils are soft enough but not mushy make two small depressions in the lentils and place the mushrooms on top of the lentils. Crack one egg over the top of each layer of mushrooms so that there are two eggs on top of the lentils.

Cook for about ten minutes. Add water to the pan 2 tablespoons at a time to keep a small amount of liquid in the bottom of the pan. Cook until the white part of the egg has set. Serve.

"The wise man puts all his eggs in one basket and watches the basket."

Andrew Carnegie, Industrialist

The refrigerator light goes on...
This is a lovely recipe that I had while in Spain. It's simple and so great for you. What is more wholesome than lentils and eggs? It is really simple and takes all of 30 minutes active cooking time.

Nutrition Facts

Serving size	about 2 cups lentils with 1 egg
Servings	2
Calories 357	Calories from Fat 112
	(% Daily Value)
Total Fat 13g	(19%)
Saturated Fat 3g	(13%)
Trans Fat 0 g	
Monounsaturated Fat 7g	
Cholesterol 211mg	(70%)
Sodium 371mg	(15%)
Total Carbohydrates 41g	(14%)
Dietary Fiber 17g	(69%)
Sugars 7g	
Protein 22g	
Vitamin A 11%	Vitamin C 19%
Calcium 8%	Iron 29%
Vitamin K 12 mcg	
Potassium 871 mg	Magnesium 82 mg

Mediterranean Tortilla

4 **45 min.**

Serving size = 1/2 pie (as a dinner meal)

This recipe keeps well for about 24 – 48 hours in the refrigerator. Makes great leftovers both cold and re-heated. This recipe can be multiplied by two but will require a larger skillet.

2 tsp	olive oil (divided)
8 ounces	red potatoes (halved)
1 small	red bell pepper
2 cloves	garlic (minced)
1 small	onion (diced)
3 large	eggs
2 large	egg whites
1/8 tsp	salt
1 Tbsp	capers
1 Tbsp	fresh oregano (minced)
1/8 tsp	red pepper flakes
to taste	fresh ground black pepper
1 small	tomato (thinly sliced into rounds)
1/2 ounce	Parmigiano-Reggiano (grated)

Preheat the oven to 325°F.

Place 1 teaspoon of the olive oil in a medium skillet. Add the potatoes and place the pan in the oven.

Place the red pepper in the oven directly on the rack (not in the pan).

Roast the potatoes, tossing occasionally, for about 30 minutes.

Roast the red bell pepper for about 30 minutes, turning at least twice.

Remove the now-blackened pepper from the oven and place in a small paper bag to cool. Remove the potatoes from the oven and place on a plate. Set aside.

When the pepper is cool, peel the skin off and seed it, then cut into strips.

In a bowl, gently whisk together the egg whites, egg yolks, salt, capers, oregano, red pepper flakes and fresh ground pepper. Fold together gently until well blended.

Heat the remaining 1 teaspoon olive oil (in the same skillet in which you roasted the potatoes) over medium-high heat and add the garlic. Cook for about one minute. Add the onions and cook for about 4 minutes, stirring frequently, until the onions are translucent but not browned. Add the potatoes and peppers. Toss.

Remove the pan from the heat and pour the egg mixture over the garlic, onions, potatoes and peppers.

Layer the sliced tomato over the top of the eggs in a circular pattern (as if it were a pizza). Place the pan in the oven and bake for about 20 minutes.

Remove and sprinkle the cheese over the top of the tomatoes. Place the pan back in the oven for about 2 minutes.

Remove and let cool for one minute, then serve.

The refrigerator light goes on...
"Tortilla" is the Spanish word for "little cake" and in Spain tortillas are baked egg dishes like this one. They are so quick and easy and make for a perfect quick evening dish. Fill them with veggies and you have a complete meal in a single pan.

Nutrition Facts

Serving size	1/2 pie
Servings	2
Calories 336	Calories from Fat 130
	(% Daily Value)
Total Fat 14g	(22%)
Saturated Fat 4g	(16%)
Trans Fat 0 g	
Monounsaturated Fat 7g	
Cholesterol 322mg	(109%)
Sodium 477mg	(20%)
Total Carbohydrates 33g	(13%)
Dietary Fiber 4g	(21%)
Sugars 9g	
Protein 21g	
Vitamin A 54%	Vitamin C 170%
Calcium 19%	Iron 16%
Vitamin K 14 mcg	
Potassium 1020 mg	Magnesium 61 mg

Mushroom Risotto

3 **45 min.**

Serving size = about 2 cups

This recipe can easily be multiplied by 2, 3, 4 or 5. This keeps well for a day or so in the refrigerator. Reheat gently. Serve with Zucchini Salad or Jicama Slaw (included).

1 tsp	extra virgin olive oil
3 cloves	garlic (minced)
1 small	white onion (diced)
1/4 lb	button mushrooms (sliced)
1 cup	arborio rice
1/4 cup	white wine
2 cups	water
1/8 tsp	salt
to taste	fresh ground black pepper
2 ounces	wild mushrooms (morels, crimini, shiitake or oyster) (sliced)
1 Tbsp	(per serving) fresh basil (chiffonade)
1 1/2 ounces	Parmigiano-Reggiano (grated)
2 medium	tomatoes (seeded and diced)

Heat the olive oil over medium-heat in a medium sized stock-pot. Add the minced garlic and cook slowly. Do not allow to brown.

When the garlic is soft and translucent, add the onions and cook until they are also translucent. Add the button mushrooms and cook over medium-high heat until they begin to turn brown. Continue to cook, stirring continuously until the mushrooms are a dark roasted brown.

Add the risotto and cook for about 2 minutes, stirring frequently.

Reduce the heat to medium and add the white wine . Stir well. Cook for one minute and add 2 cups of water, the salt and pepper.

Cook over medium-heat, stirring frequently so that the rice will not stick to the bottom. After about 15 minutes, check to see if the rice is done. Add more water, 1/4 cup at a time as needed.

Slice the wild mushrooms.

When the rice is soft but not mushy, add the basil, wild mushrooms and parmesan cheese. Stir and cook for another 2 - 3 minutes over very low heat.

Serve topped with the julienne tomatoes.

"We are indeed much more than what we eat, but what we eat can nevertheless help us to be much more than what we are."

Adelle Davis, Nutritionist

The refrigerator light goes on...
Cooking mushrooms is not a timid enterprise. Because they are mostly water, mushrooms must be cooked until they begin to caramelize to bring out their rich flavor.

Nutrition Facts

Serving size	about 2 cups
Servings	3
Calories 373	Calories from Fat 54
	(% Daily Value)
Total Fat 6g	(9%)
Saturated Fat 3g	(14%)
Trans Fat 0 g	
Monounsaturated Fat 2g	
Cholesterol 12mg	(4%)
Sodium 326mg	(14%)
Total Carbohydrates 63g	(21%)
Dietary Fiber 4g	(15%)
Sugars 4g	
Protein 12g	
Vitamin A 18%	Vitamin C 23%
Calcium 24%	Iron 20%
Vitamin K 19 mcg	
Potassium 585 mg	Magnesium 42 mg

Mushroom Souffle

2 **30 min.**

Serving size = 1 souffle

This recipe can be multiplied. No leftovers: eat it while you can.

4 ounces	wild type mushrooms (oyster, shiitake, crimini)
1/4 cup	sherry
2 Tbsp	balsamic vinegar
1/8	red bell pepper (slice into julienne strips)
2 ounces	low-fat Swiss cheese (shredded fine)
3/4 cup	2% milk
1 large	egg yolk
1/4 cup	all purpose white flour
1/2 tsp	unsalted butter
3 large	egg whites
1	tomato (peeled and chopped)
4	leaves fresh basil (chiffonade)

Heat a small, non-stick sauté pan over high medium-high heat and add the mushrooms, sherry and balsamic vinegar. Cook over high heat, tossing occasionally. When the mushrooms are cooked, add the peppers. Continue to reduce until no liquid is left. Set aside.

In a blender, place Swiss cheese, milk, egg yolk and flour. Blend until smooth.

Preheat the oven to 400°F.

Butter two soufflé dishes. Divide the mushroom and pepper mixture evenly and place in the bottom of the soufflé dishes.

Whisk the egg whites in a copper bowl until they form stiff peaks. Fold together with the cheese mixture carefully.

Divide the soufflé mixture evenly between the two soufflé dishes on top of the mushroom mixture.

Place in the oven and reduce the heat to 375°F. Bake for about 10 minutes, until puffed and slightly browned on top.

While this is cooking, combine the tomato and basil.

Serve immediately with the tomato-basil mixture.

"The only thing that will make a soufflé fall is if it knows you are afraid of it."

James Beard, Father of
American Cuisine

The refrigerator light goes on...
Healthy recipe tip: Combining the flour and milk with the cheese makes a thick sauce that doesn't need extra fat.

If you don't have a copper bowl, add a pinch of cream of tartar to the egg white to help form stiff peaks.

Nutrition Facts

Serving size	1 souffle
Servings	2
Calories 346	Calories from Fat 117
	(% Daily Value)
Total Fat 13g	(18%)
Saturated Fat 7g	(35%)
Trans Fat 0 g	
Monounsaturated Fat n/a g	
Cholesterol 135mg	(45%)
Sodium 212mg	(9%)
Total Carbohydrates 27g	(9%)
Dietary Fiber 2g	(8%)
Sugars n/a g	
Protein 22g	
Vitamin A 54%	Vitamin C 113%
Calcium 44%	Iron 13%
Vitamin K 10 mcg	
Potassium 782 mg	Magnesium 48 mg

Parmesan Gnocchi

2 **45 min.**

Serving size = 10-15 gnocchi

This recipe can easily be multiplied up to 8 times. Leftovers are fair at best. I have kept the uncooked gnocchi refrigerated overnight but they are not as good as when fresh.

Serve with the sauce from Fettuccine Alfredo, with Dill Pesto, or with Tomato Sauce, and also with Roasted Beets or Parmesan Squash or Green Beans in Walnut Vinaigrette (recipes included).

10 ounces	Yukon Gold potatoes
2 Tbsp	all purpose white flour
1 ounce	Parmigiano-Reggiano
3 Tbsp	whole wheat flour
1 large	egg
1/4 tsp	salt
1/8 tsp	ground black pepper
4 quarts	water

Place a steamer basket in a large sauce pan. Add about 1 1/2 cups water and set the pan over high heat. Steam the cubed potatoes until very tender (about 20 minutes). Remove the steamer basket and allow the potatoes to cool until they are no more than warm to the touch.

Force all of the steamed potatoes through a potato ricer into a large mixing bowl. (If you don't have a potato ricer, the potatoes must be chopped until there are no lumps. Do not over mash them or the gnocchi will be pasty.)

Add the all purpose flour and the parmesan cheese to the potatoes with the egg, salt and black pepper. Mix together using a fork. The mixture will take on a crumbly consistency. Add 1 tablespoon of whole wheat flour and blend well.

Knead the dough gently until all the flour is blended in. Stop kneading when the flour is incorporated.

After the dough is smooth, cut it into 2 equal pieces. Place two tablespoons of the whole wheat flour on a cutting board and roll each piece of dough into a rope about as big around as your thumb.

Cut the ropes in 1/2 inch pieces (about ten per roll) and then roll the dumpling over the tines of a fork to shape the ridges of the gnocchi.

Boil at least 4 quarts of water and add the gnocchi no more than 2 servings at a time (20 gnocchi).

As they float to the top of the water, they are done. Remove them and add to prepared sauce.

"Not presume to dictate, but broiled fowl and mushrooms - capital thing!"
Charles Dickens, Author

The refrigerator light goes on...
This recipe is a little richer than some of the other Dr. Gourmet gnocchi recipes. The parmesan adds a smooth and creamy flavor that goes well with almost any sauce. The flavor's so rich and sweet that they almost don't need any sauce, but they are perfect with a fresh tomato sauce.

Nutrition Facts

Serving size	10-15 gnocchi
Servings	2

Calories 279	Calories from Fat 58
	(% Daily Value)
Total Fat 7g	(10%)
Saturated Fat 3g	(16%)
Trans Fat 0 g	
Monounsaturated Fat 2 g	
Cholesterol 115mg	(38%)
Sodium 558mg	(23%)
Total Carbohydrates 43g	(14%)
Dietary Fiber 4g	(17%)
Sugars 2 g	
Protein 13g	
Vitamin A 4%	Vitamin C 17%
Calcium 20%	Iron 10%
Vitamin K 4 mcg	
Potassium 551 mg	Magnesium 65 mg

Penne with Eggplant Pesto and Mushrooms

2 **30 min.**

Serving size = 2 ounces pasta with sauce

This recipe can easily be multiplied and requires making Eggplant Pesto (recipe included). This recipe does not make very good leftovers.

3 quarts	water
4 ounces	whole wheat penne
1 tsp	olive oil
16 ounces	crimini mushrooms (sliced)
1 large	onion (sliced)
1/2	recipe Eggplant Pesto
1	bottled roasted red pepper (thinly sliced)

Place the water in a large stock pot over high heat. When the water boils add the pasta.

While the water is heating and the pasta is boiling place a large skillet over medium heat. Add the olive oil and mushrooms. Cook, stirring occasionally, until the mushrooms begin to turn dark brown and caramelize.

Add the onions after about 5 minutes and cook for 5 – 7 minutes until the onions begin to turn soft.

As the penne is nearing being done add the pesto and pepper to the pan and toss until the pesto is warm. Add the penne. If the sauce is too thick, add a small amount of the pasta water.

Serve.

"When I was alone, I lived on eggplant, the stove top cook's strongest ally...."

Laurie Colwin, Cookbook Author

The refrigerator light goes on...
Pestos are super versatile and this eggplant pesto goes great with so many combinations. You can use almost whatever you have in the kitchen as leftovers – veggies, a little ham, some grated parmesan – almost anything will make a great meal in a flash.

Nutrition Facts

Serving size	2 ounces pasta with sauce
Servings	2
Calories 501	Calories from Fat 148
	(% Daily Value)
Total Fat 17g	(27%)
Saturated Fat 3g	(15%)
Trans Fat 0 g	
Monounsaturated Fat 5 g	
Cholesterol 5mg	(2%)
Sodium 284mg	(12%)
Total Carbohydrates 73g	(24%)
Dietary Fiber 13g	(53%)
Sugars 13 g	
Protein 21g	
Vitamin A 21%	Vitamin C 83%
Calcium 20%	Iron 23%
Vitamin K 15 mcg	
Potassium 1686 mg	Magnesium 158 mg

Penne with Roasted Acorn Squash

2 **60 min.**

Serving size = 2 ounces pasta with veggies

This recipe can easily be multiplied but does not make good leftovers.

	spray oil
1	acorn squash (halved and seeded)
3 quarts	water
4 ounces	whole wheat penne pasta
2 tsp	olive oil
2	ribs celery (sliced crosswise)
1 large	shallot (peeled and sliced thinly)
2 Tbsp	pinenuts
1/8 tsp	salt
to taste	fresh ground black pepper
1/4 cup	white wine
1 ounce	arugula
3 ounces	smoked gouda cheese (shredded)

Preheat oven to 325°F. Spray a large skillet lightly with oil. Place the acorn squash halves in the skillet, cut side down. Place the pan in the oven and roast for 30 minutes. Remove and let cool in pan.

When the squash is cool cut 1/2 of it into large 3/4 inch cubes. (Put the other half in the fridge for another use.)

Place the water in a large sauce pan over high heat. When the water is boiling, add the penne pasta.

While the pasta is cooking, place a large non-stick skillet over medium heat. Add the celery, shallots and pinenuts. Cook, stirring frequently, for about 10 minutes. Adjust the heat so that none of the ingredients brown, but cook gently.

When the pasta is done, drain, but reserve 1 cup of the cooking water. Add the drained pasta to the skillet with the shallots and celery. Add the white wine, salt and pepper and toss well.

Increase the heat to medium-high. Cook, tossing frequently, for about 3 minutes. Add the pasta water 1/4 cup at a time to help create a sauce. (You may only need about 1/2 cup.)

Add the cubed squash and arugula. Cook for one minute. Add the smoked gouda and cook for about a minute until the cheese is melted. Serve.

"Take the obvious, add a cupful of brains, a generous pinch of imagination, a bucketful of courage and daring, stir well and bring to a boil."
Barnard Baruch, Economist

The refrigerator light goes on...
Acorn squash means Fall to me. This is a great savory dish that's warm and comforting for those cool fall evenings. Note that it uses only half of the acorn squash, leaving the other half for recipes or a fine lunch.

Nutrition Facts

Serving size	2 ounces pasta with veggies
Servings	2
Calories 538	Calories from Fat 198
	(% Daily Value)
Total Fat 23g	(35%)
Saturated Fat 9g	(43%)
Trans Fat 0 g	
Monounsaturated Fat 8 g	
Cholesterol 48mg	(16%)
Sodium 538mg	(22%)
Total Carbohydrates 63g	(21%)
Dietary Fiber 7g	(30%)
Sugars 3 g	
Protein 22g	
Vitamin A 30%	Vitamin C 29%
Calcium 40%	Iron 23%
Vitamin K 35 mcg	
Potassium 866 mg	Magnesium 168 mg

Portobello Burgers

1 **30 min.**

Serving size = 1 burger

This recipe can easily be multiplied but does not make good leftovers.

Serve with one of the following: Thick Cut Yam Fries, Parsnip French Fries, or French Fries (recipes included).

	spray olive oil
1	3 ounce Portobello mushroom cap
2 Tbsp	barbecue sauce (low sodium if possible)
1 ounce	provolone cheese (sliced)
1 small	tomato (2 slices per burger)
1 small	onion (2 slices per burger)
2	leaves lettuce
to taste	fresh ground black pepper
1	whole wheat hamburger bun

Place a large skillet in the oven and preheat to 425°F.

When the oven is hot spray the pan lightly with oil and place the mushroom with the top down. Spread the barbecue sauce over the gills of the mushroom.

Cook for about 5 minutes and then turn over. Cook for another 5 minutes and turn one more time.

If you like your bun toasted place it on the rack in the oven.

After two minutes remove the bun and place the mushroom on the bottom half. Top with the tomato, onion, lettuce, black pepper and the top of the bun.

"Falling in love is like eating mushrooms: you never know if it's the real thing until it's too late."
Bill Balance, Radio personality

The refrigerator light goes on...
It simply doesn't get easier than this to make dinner. Put the mushroom in the oven with some barbecue sauce on it, turn, turn, serve.

I've had a lot of Portobello mushroom "burgers" at restaurants here and there. They're good, and even though mushrooms are one of the pure umami flavors, there's always seemed to be something missing. Credit to my wife for suggesting the barbecue sauce. It adds just the right touch.

If you are watching your sodium there are low-sodium barbecue sauces on the market. I have also been seeing more and more bottled sauces that are not made with high fructose corn syrup. While these do use sugar instead, it's not a lot, and two tablespoons is only about 50 calories.

Nutrition Facts

Serving size	2 ounces pasta with sauce
Servings	2
Calories 501	Calories from Fat 148
	(% Daily Value)
Total Fat 17g	(27%)
Saturated Fat 3g	(15%)
Trans Fat 0 g	
Monounsaturated Fat 5 g	
Cholesterol 5mg	(2%)
Sodium 284mg	(12%)
Total Carbohydrates 73g	(24%)
Dietary Fiber 13g	(53%)
Sugars 13 g	
Protein 21g	
Vitamin A 21%	Vitamin C 83%
Calcium 20%	Iron 23%
Vitamin K 15 mcg	
Potassium 1686 mg	Magnesium 158 mg

Quick and Easy Tomato Sauce and Pasta

6 **30 min.**

Serving size = 3/4 cup sauce with 2 ounces pasta and 1/2 ounce cheese

This recipe can be multiplied and makes great leftovers.

1 Tbsp	olive oil
3 cloves	garlic (sliced)
1 large	onion (diced)
1 1/2 lbs	Roma tomatoes (quartered)
2 cups	water
1/2 tsp	salt
to taste	fresh ground black pepper
1 Tbsp	dried basil
1 tsp	dried oregano
4 quarts	water
12 ounces	whole wheat pasta
3 ounces	parmesan cheese (grated)

Place the olive oil in a large skillet over medium-high heat. Add the garlic and onions. Cook for about 5 minutes, stirring frequently.

Add the tomatoes and cook for about 5 minutes, stirring frequently.

Add the water, salt, pepper, basil and oregano.

Reduce the heat to medium so that the sauce is simmering. Cook for about 15 – 20 minutes, stirring occasionally.

While the sauce is cooking place the water on to boil. After it is at a full boil add the pasta and cook, stirring occasionally, until al dente. Drain and then top with about 3/4 cup sauce and 1/2 ounce cheese.

"I want to go back to Brazil, get married, have lots of kids, and just be a couch tomato."
Ana Barros, Model

The refrigerator light goes on...
Proof positive that eating healthy is easy, delicious and also inexpensive. This recipe serves 6 and with 2 ounces whole wheat pasta and 3 tablespoons of cheese per serving it's only about 75 cents each. That's it. The ingredients for a meal that serves six cost about 5 dollars. Healthy, easy, delicious and smart.

Nutrition Facts

Serving size	3/4 cup sauce with 2 ounces pasta and 1/2 ounce cheese
Servings	2
Calories 298	Calories from Fat 60
	(% Daily Value)
Total Fat 7g	(11%)
Saturated Fat 3g	(14%)
Trans Fat 0 g	
Monounsaturated Fat 3 g	
Cholesterol 10mg	(3%)
Sodium 429mg	(18%)
Total Carbohydrates 49	(16%)
Dietary Fiber 6g	(25%)
Sugars 4 g	
Protein 14g	
Vitamin A 21%	Vitamin C 27%
Calcium 21%	Iron 15%
Vitamin K 17 mcg	
Potassium 430 mg	Magnesium 101 mg

Quick Tacos

2 ⏱ **30 min.**

Serving size = 3 tacos

This recipe can easily be multiplied. The filling for the tacos will keep well for a few days in the refrigerator.

1 15 ounce can	no salt added diced tomatoes
1/2 tsp	ground cumin
1/4 tsp	paprika
1/2 tsp	dried oregano
1/4 tsp	chili powder
1/8 tsp	red pepper flakes (optional)
1/4 tsp	salt
to taste	fresh ground black pepper
1 cup	no salt added frozen corn kernels
6	taco shells (trans fat free)
3 ounces	reduced-fat cheddar or Monterey Jack cheese

Place the diced tomatoes in a medium skillet over medium heat.

Add the cumin, paprika, oregano, chili powder, red pepper flakes, salt and pepper. Cook, stirring occasionally, for about 15 minutes.

As the tomatoes cook, the liquid will reduce and the tomatoes will thicken. At that point add the corn and cook for about 3 - 5 minutes.

Divide the grated cheese into two small piles. Using one pile place a small amount of cheese in the bottom of each taco shell, dividing the cheese evenly between the 6 tacos.

Add equal amounts of the tomato and corn mixture to the 6 tacos.

Top the taco filling with the remaining cheese, divided evenly between the 6 tacos. Serve.

"Even the most resourceful housewife cannot create miracles from a riceless pantry."
Chinese Proverb

The refrigerator light goes on...
The idea of Dr. Gourmet Pantry Meals™ is that you'll have items in your pantry or 'fridge that can be quickly put together for a great meal. Use recipes such as these tacos as a guide. If you have an onion, it's easy to dice it and add to the tomatoes instead of the corn, for instance. Have some fresh lettuce or cilantro on hand? That'll go well also. The key is to have the fundamentals in the house that you can use to make a quick healthy meal.

Do keep in mind that many of the most popular taco shells on the market, including Old El Paso, still contain trans fats (amazing in this day and age). Check the package and purchase only those that don't have any trans fats. Brands I have seen without trans fats include Taco Bell (made by Kraft) and Casa Fiesta.

Nutrition Facts

Serving size	3 tacos
Servings	2

Calories 309	Calories from Fat 93
	(% Daily Value)
Total Fat 10g	(16%)
Saturated Fat 3g	(17%)
Trans Fat 0 g	
Monounsaturated Fat 5 g	
Cholesterol 9mg	(3%)
Sodium 687mg	(29%)
Total Carbohydrates 41g	(14%)
Dietary Fiber 5g	(19%)
Sugars 5 g	
Protein 16g	
Vitamin A 12%	Vitamin C 20%
Calcium 25%	Iron 15%
Vitamin K 8 mcg	
Potassium 494 mg	Magnesium 71 mg

Quinoa Caprese Salad

4 **30 min.**

Serving size = about 2 cups salad

This recipe can be multiplied. This recipe is great the second day and will keep about 48 hours in the fridge.

2 cups	water
1 cup	quinoa
1 small	shallot (minced)
1 medium	zucchini (diced)
1 large	rib celery (diced)
1/2 medium	green pepper (diced)
8 ounces	grape tomatoes (sliced in half lengthwise)
8 small	black olives (thinly sliced)
8 ounces	fresh mozzarella (cut into 1/2 inch dice)
3 Tbsp	olive oil
4 tsp	white wine vinegar
1/2 tsp	salt
to taste	fresh ground black pepper
8	leaves fresh basil (chiffonade)

Place the water in a medium sauce pan over high heat. When the water boils, add the quinoa.

Reduce the heat to a simmer. Stir occasionally. The quinoa will take about 20 minutes to cook. When the water is gone, the quinoa is done. Place the cooked quinoa in a large mixing bowl and refrigerate until cool.

When the quinoa is cool, add the zucchini, celery, pepper, tomatoes, olives, mozzarella, olive oil, vinegar, salt, pepper and basil.

Fold together until well blended. Chill, then serve.

"Cheese - milk's leap toward immortality."
Clifton Fadiman, Author

The refrigerator light goes on...
This may be the best salad ever. OK, that's a bit hyperbolic but, still, it's really, really good. The classic caprese salad (in the style of Capri) using mozzarella, tomato and basil was the inspiration for this recipe. To make a complete meal and add a bit of body I tossed in the other veggies and the vinaigrette. As I was working on this I thought that it would be good, but this is a lot better than good. The caprese flavors come through with a bit of a twist and the textures of the veggies and cheese with the quinoa is perfect. Take this one to your next pot luck.

Nutrition Facts

Serving size	about 2 cups salad
Servings	4
Calories 455	Calories from Fat 230
	(% Daily Value)
Total Fat 26g	(40%)
Saturated Fat 9g	(46%)
Trans Fat 0 g	
Monounsaturated Fat 12 g	
Cholesterol 44mg	(15%)
Sodium 719mg	(30%)
Total Carbohydrates 36g	(12%)
Dietary Fiber 5g	(20%)
Sugars 4 g	
Protein 20g	
Vitamin A 26%	Vitamin C 48%
Calcium 34%	Iron 17%
Vitamin K 24 mcg	
Potassium 663 mg	Magnesium 117 mg

Roasted Southwestern Acorn Squash

2 45 min.

Serving size = 1 filled squash

This recipe can easily be multiplied but does not make very good leftovers.

1 large	acorn squash (halved and seeded)
1 tsp	olive oil
1 clove	garlic (minced)
1 small	onion (diced)
1	rib celery (diced)
1 small	carrot (peeled and diced)
1 15 ounce can	no salt added black beans (drained and rinsed)
1/2 tsp	ground cumin
1/2 tsp	chili powder
1/4 tsp	salt
to taste	fresh ground black pepper
1 small	red bell pepper (seeded and diced)
1/4 cup	cilantro leaves
3 ounces	Monterey jack cheese (shredded)

Preheat the oven to 375°F. Place the acorn squash halves cut side down on a cookie sheet or a large skillet and roast in the oven for about 30 minutes until tender.

While the squash is roasting place the olive oil in a large skillet over medium-high heat. Add the garlic and onions and cook for about 3 - 4 minutes. Add the celery and carrots and cook for another 3 - 4 minutes.

Add the black beans, cumin, chili powder, salt, pepper and diced red pepper. Toss well and cook for about 3 - 4 minutes. Remove from the heat until the squash are finished roasting.

When the squash is roasted spoon the black bean mixture equally into the halves. Top the squash with the shredded cheese and return to the oven for about 5 - 10 minutes until the cheese is melted.

"You know, when you get your first asparagus, or your first acorn squash, or your first really good tomato of the season, those are the moments that define the cook's year. I get more excited by that than anything else."

Mario Batali, Chef

The refrigerator light goes on...
Roasted acorn squash is fantastic and so versatile. It makes the perfect side dish but this is a simple and delicious way to get everything good for you in a main course. Beans, veggies, high fiber, great vitamins... You won't even know that it's good for you.

Nutrition Facts

Serving size	1 filled squash
Servings	2
Calories 462	Calories from Fat 114
	(% Daily Value)
Total Fat 13g	(20%)
Saturated Fat 7g	(33%)
Trans Fat 0 g	
Monounsaturated Fat 4 g	
Cholesterol 27mg	(9%)
Sodium 583mg	(24%)
Total Carbohydrates 65g	(22%)
Dietary Fiber 18g	(71%)
Sugars 6 g	
Protein 27g	
Vitamin A 149%	Vitamin C 41%
Calcium 44%	Iron 30%
Vitamin K 21 mcg	
Potassium 1579 mg	Magnesium 190 mg

Spaghetti with Zucchini and Tomatoes

2 **30 min.**

Serving size = 2 ounces pasta with vegetables

This recipe can easily be multiplied. This recipe makes fair leftovers. Reheat gently.

2 medium	tomatoes (peeled, seeded and chopped)
3 quarts	water
1 Tbsp	olive oil
1 clove	garlic
1 large	shallot (minced)
2 large	zucchini (diced)
4	fresh sage leaves (or 1 Tbsp. dried)
1/8 tsp	dried tarragon
2 1/2 ounces	fresh mozzarella (diced)
1 1/2 ounces	Parmigiano-Reggiano (grated)
4 ounces	whole wheat spaghetti

Place the water in a large stock pot over high heat.

To peel the tomatoes, as the water comes to a boil reduce the heat to medium. Drop the whole tomato in the pot of water. After about 90 seconds, remove it and place the tomato on the counter. When it is cooled the skin will easily slip off. Discard the skin and seeds and chop the tomatoes.

Leave the pot on the stove as that water can be used to cook the pasta.

Place a large skillet over medium high heat. Add the olive oil and the whole clove of garlic with the minced shallot. Cook, stirring frequently for about 3 - 5 minutes. Add the diced zucchini, sage and tarragon.

Cook over medium to medium-high heat for about 10 minutes and add the chopped tomato. Toss frequently.

When you add the tomato bring the pasta water back to a boil. Add the spaghetti. Stir the pasta occasionally.

Add the mozzarella to the zucchini and toss. As it begins to melt add the Parmigiano-reggiano.

Toss the vegetables together with the cheese, and as the spaghetti is done, drain it and place it in the skillet. Toss the pasta with the vegetables. Remove the whole garlic clove and serve.

"As long as there's pasta and Chinese food in the world, I'm okay."

Michael Chang, Tennis Pro

The refrigerator light goes on...
Even if you don't think you like zucchini, this is a great dish. It is so sweet and savory and rich and creamy. It's almost the perfect winter pasta – quick, easy and warming.

Nutrition Facts

Serving size	2 ounces pasta with vegetables
Servings	2
Calories 506	Calories from Fat 188
	(% Daily Value)
Total Fat 21g	(33%)
Saturated Fat 9g	(46%)
Trans Fat 0 g	
Monounsaturated Fat 9 g	
Cholesterol 41mg	(14%)
Sodium 588mg	(25%)
Total Carbohydrates 57g	(19%)
Dietary Fiber 8g	(34%)
Sugars 7 g	
Protein 27g	
Vitamin A 38%	Vitamin C 84%
Calcium 50%	Iron 20%
Vitamin K 28 mcg	
Potassium 1021 mg	Magnesium 147 mg

Tamale Pie with Black Beans

6 **30 min.**

Serving size = about 2 cups

This recipe can be multiplied, but you should use separate pans. This recipe makes good leftovers.

1 tsp	olive oil
2 cloves	garlic (minced)
1	10 ounce package frozen diced onions
1	10 ounce package mixed peppers (or chopped green peppers)
1 15 ounce can	no salt added diced tomatoes
1 tsp	ground cumin
1/2 tsp	chili powder
1/2 tsp	salt
2 15 ounce cans	no salt added black beans (drained and rinsed)
	spray oil
8	taco shells
8 ounces	reduced-fat Monterey jack cheese (shredded)

Preheat the oven to 375°F.

Place the oil in a large skillet over medium-high heat. Add the minced garlic while the pan is heating, stirring frequently.

When the pan is hot add the onions and peppers. Cook for about 5 minutes, stirring frequently.

Add the tomatoes, cumin, chili powder and salt and cook for 10 minutes. Stir occasionally.

Fold the beans into the tomato mixture.

Lightly coat a 10 inch oblong pan with the cooking spray. Add 1/3 of the tomato bean mixture to the bottom of the pan. Top with a layer of 4 of the taco shells broken in half to lie flat.

Add another 1/3 of the tomato bean mixture on top of the taco shells. Top this with 1/3 of the cheese. Top with a layer of 4 of the taco shells broken in half to lie flat.

Add the final 1/3 of the tomato bean mixture on top

of the taco shells. Top this with the remaining cheese.

Bake in the preheated oven for 15 minutes.

"Never order food in excess of your body weight."
Erma Bombeck, Housewife

The refrigerator light goes on...
Growing up this had a lot of names depending on whose house I was at. Tortilla casserole, taco casserole, tamale pie, it didn't matter. And there are endless variations. This one was created to be as simple as possible and to use items out of your pantry or freezer.

This is also made to be more family friendly and is less spicy than some folks might want. A bit more cumin (an extra teaspoon) and chili powder (another 1/2 teaspoon) will give it more flavor. Adding a bit of cayenne pepper adds the zing that you might crave.

Nutrition Facts

Serving size	about 2 cups
Servings	6

Calories 356	Calories from Fat 117
	(% Daily Value)
Total Fat 13g	(20%)
Saturated Fat 6g	(21%)
Trans Fat 0 g	
Monounsaturated Fat 5 g	
Cholesterol 24mg	(8%)
Sodium 482mg	(20%)
Total Carbohydrates 41g	(14%)
Dietary Fiber 11g	(42%)
Sugars 5 g	
Protein 21g	
Vitamin A 10%	Vitamin C 78%
Calcium 34%	Iron 19%
Vitamin K 8 mcg	
Potassium 649 mg	Magnesium 102 mg

Tomato and White Bean Soup

4 **75 min.**

Serving size = about 2 cups

This recipe can easily be multiplied up to 8 times. Keeps well for 2-4 days in the refrigerator. Reheat in the microwave for 1 minute loosely covered, stir, then heat another minute.

2 tsp	olive oil
2 large	white onions (large dice)
4 large	ribs celery (large dice)
2 15 ounce cans	no salt added diced tomatoes
2 15 ounce cans	no salt added cannellini beans (NOT drained and rinsed)
2 cups	water
1/2 tsp	dried marjoram
1 tsp	dried oregano
1/2 tsp	dried rosemary
1/2 tsp	salt
to taste	fresh ground black pepper
4 ounces	goat cheese

Place the olive oil in a medium stock pot or 4 quart sauce pan over medium heat.

Add the onion and celery and cook for about 7 to 8 minutes. Stir frequently.

Add the tomatoes, beans (with liquid), water, marjoram, oregano, rosemary, salt and pepper.

Bring the soup to a simmer and reduce the heat to a slow simmer. Cook for about 45 minutes. Stir occasionally.

Remove the soup from the heat, stir and let cool for about 5 minutes. Add the goat cheese and stir until melted.

Serve.

"Good intentions are not enough. They've never put an onion in the soup yet."
Sonya Levien, Screenwriter

The refrigerator light goes on...
Soups that are chunky and full of body are great for a cold weather meal. Filling, warming and so satisfying. The key for this soup is cutting the veggies in a large dice and using larger white beans like the cannellini. Slow simmering softens the beans and veggies and adds to the creamy texture..

Nutrition Facts

Serving size	about 2 cups
Servings	6
Calories 366	Calories from Fat 82
	(% Daily Value)
Total Fat 8g	(14%)
Saturated Fat 4g	(19%)
Trans Fat 0 g	
Monounsaturated Fat 3 g	
Cholesterol 13mg	(4%)
Sodium 458mg	(18%)
Total Carbohydrates 53g	(17%)
Dietary Fiber 13g	(45%)
Sugars 10 g	
Protein 20g	
Vitamin A 13%	Vitamin C 42%
Calcium 28%	Iron 42%
Vitamin K 26 mcg	
Potassium 1374 mg	Magnesium 126 mg

Tortellini Primavera

2 **30 min.**

Serving size =about 2 cups

This recipe can easily be multiplied by up to 8 times, but does not make good leftovers.

3 quarts	water
4 ounces	tortellini
1 Tbsp	olive oil
1 large	shallot (minced)
1 clove	garlic (minced)
1 large	carrot (peeled and diced)
1 large	yellow squash (seeded and diced)
2/3 cup	frozen, shelled fava beans (thawed)
1 medium	tomato (seeded and diced)
1 ounce	goat cheese (crumbled)
1/4 tsp	salt
to taste	fresh ground black pepper
4 large	basil leaves (chiffonade)

"Spring is nature's way of saying, 'Let's party!'"
Robin Williams, Comedian

The refrigerator light goes on...
Primavera stems from the Latin *primus* meaning first or spring. I love naming recipes that are full of veggies this way. You're not stuck with the ones in this recipe - use what is fresh if you can. Cook the firmer vegetables first and add the softer ones near the end. There are so many great substitutions - peas, zucchini - whatever strikes your fancy.

Place the water in a large stock pot over high heat.

When the water boils add the tortellini. Stir well.

While the tortellini is cooking place the olive oil in a large skillet over medium-high heat. Add the shallot, garlic and carrot. Cook, stirring frequently, for about 5 - 8 minutes.

Add the fava beans and the tomatoes. Toss and cook for about 2 minutes. If the tortellini is not done, reduce the heat to low.

When the tortellini is done reserve about 1/2 cup of the pasta water and then drain the pasta and add them to the skillet with the goat cheese, salt, pepper and basil. Toss until the cheese is melted.

If the sauce is too thick, add the pasta water one tablespoon at a time until it is the desired thickness.

Nutrition Facts

Serving size	about 2 cups
Servings	2
Calories 428	Calories from Fat 153
	(% Daily Value)
Total Fat 17g	(27%)
Saturated Fat 7g	(36%)
Trans Fat 0 g	
Monounsaturated Fat 8 g	
Cholesterol 36mg	(12%)
Sodium 622mg	(26%)
Total Carbohydrates 51g	(17%)
Dietary Fiber 7g	(28%)
Sugars 5 g	
Protein 19g	
Vitamin A 147%	Vitamin C 29%
Calcium 19%	Iron 18%
Vitamin K 21 mcg	
Potassium 692 mg	Magnesium 71 mg

Yam Gnocchi

2 **45 min.**

Serving size = 10 gnocchi

This recipe can easily be multiplied. Leftovers are fair at best. I have kept the uncooked gnocchi refrigerated overnight but they are not as good as when fresh.

Serve with the sauce from Fettuccine Alfredo, with Dill Pesto, or with Tomato Sauce, and also with Roasted Beets or Parmesan Squash or Green Beans in Walnut Vinaigrette (recipes included).

10 ounces	yams
4 Tbsp	all purpose flour
2 Tbsp	whole wheat flour
1 large	egg
1/4 tsp	salt
1/8 tsp	ground nutmeg
1/8 tsp	ground black pepper
4 quarts	water

Place a steamer basket in a large sauce pan. Add about 1 1/2 cups water and set the pan over high heat. Steam the cubed yams until very tender (about 20 minutes). Remove the steamer basket and allow the yams to cool until they are no more than warm to the touch.

Force all of the steamed yams through a potato ricer into a large mixing bowl. (If you don't have a potato ricer, the yams must be chopped until there are no lumps. Do not over mash them or the gnocchi will be pasty.)

Add 3 tablespoons of the all purpose flour to the yams with the egg, salt, nutmeg and black pepper. Mix together using a fork. The mixture will take on a crumbly consistency. Add the 2 tablespoons of whole wheat flour and blend well.

Knead the dough gently until all the flour is blended in. Stop kneading when the flour is incorporated.

After the dough is smooth, cut it into 2 equal pieces. Place one tablespoon of all purpose flour on a cutting board and roll each piece of dough into a rope about as big around as your thumb.

Cut the ropes in 1/2 inch pieces (about ten per roll), and then roll the dumpling over the tines of a fork to shape the ridges of the gnocchi.

Boil at least 4 quarts of water and add the gnocchi no more than 2 servings at a time (20 gnocchi).

As they float to the top of the water, they are done. Remove them and add to prepared sauce.

"England has three sauces and three hundred and sixty religions, whereas France has three religions and three hundred and sixty sauces."
Talleyrand, French Diplomat

The refrigerator light goes on...
Gnocchi makes such a fantastic meal. The light pillows of potato are the perfect vehicle for almost any sauce. I love this version with yams because it is slightly sweet. It's great for you too, having 7 grams of fiber per serving. It's a fun recipe to get the kids involved in making.

Nutrition Facts

Serving size	10 gnocchi
Servings	2
Calories 288	Calories from Fat 27
	(% Daily Value)
Total Fat 3g	(5%)
Saturated Fat 1g	(5%)
Trans Fat 0 g	
Monounsaturated Fat 1 g	
Cholesterol 106mg	(35%)
Sodium 339mg	(14%)
Total Carbohydrates 58g	(19%)
Dietary Fiber 7g	(29%)
Sugars 1 g	
Protein 8g	
Vitamin A 6%	Vitamin C 41%
Calcium 4%	Iron 13%
Vitamin K 4 mcg	
Potassium 1245 mg	Magnesium 47 mg

Zucchini Chevre Risotto

2 | **30 min.**

Serving size = about 2 cups

This recipe can easily be multiplied. This keeps well for about 48 hours in the fridge. Reheat gently.

1 lb	zucchini
spray olive oil	
1 tsp	extra virgin olive oil
1 cloves	garlic
1 medium	onion
1/2 cup	arborio rice
1/4 cup	low sodium chicken or vegetable broth
2 cups	water
1/8 tsp	salt
1 tsp	fresh rosemary
1 ounce	semi-soft goat cheese
1 ounce	Pecorino-Romano cheese
to taste	fresh ground black pepper

Place a large non-stick skillet in the oven and preheat to 375°F. When the pan is hot add the diced zucchini and spray lightly with olive oil. Toss and return the pan to the oven. About every 7 minutes remove the pan and toss the zucchini carefully. After about 20 minutes the zucchini cubes should be lightly browned.

While the zucchini is cooking heat the olive oil over medium-heat in a medium sized stock-pot. Add the minced garlic and cook slowly. Do not allow to brown.

When the garlic is soft and translucent, add the onions and cook until they are also translucent.

Add the risotto and cook for about 2 minutes, stirring frequently.

Reduce the heat to medium and add the chicken stock . Stir well. Cook for one minute and add 2 cups of water the salt and rosemary.

Cook over medium-heat, stirring occasionaly so that the rice will not stick to the bottom. After about 15 minutes, check to see if the rice is done. Add more water, 1/4 cup at a time as needed.

Add the cooked zucchini when the rice is soft but not

mushy. Add the goat cheese and parmesan cheese. Stir and cook for another minute over very low heat. Season with pepper to taste.

"Zucchini
Looking for Zucchini?
Find exactly what you want today."

The refrigerator light goes on...
I love the combination of goat cheese and zucchini. The sweetness of the zucchini and the soft creamy yet slightly tart goat cheese just seem meant for each other. I get a number of emails about substitutions for goat cheese and I try to convince people to use goat cheeses in recipes such as this. While it may be a bit of an acquired taste, once you have you'll be using goat cheeses all the time.

Nutrition Facts

Serving Size	about 2 cups
Servings	2

Calories 359	Calories from Fat 87
	(% Daily Value)
Total Fat 10 g	(15 %)
Saturated Fat 5 g	(25 %)
Trans Fat 0 g	
Monounsaturated Fat 4 g	
Cholesterol 21 mg	(8 %)
Sodium 394 mg	(16 %)
Total Carbohydrates 55 g	(18 %)
Dietary Fiber 5 g	(20 %)
Sugars 7 g	
Protein 14 g	
Vitamin A 17 %	Vitamin C 43 %
Calcium 21 %	Iron 19 %
Vitamin K 12 mcg	
Potassium 766 mg	Magnesium 55 mg

Made in the USA
Coppell, TX
11 February 2022

73318557R00057